LIVE LONGER
LOOK YOUNGER

This book is dedicated to my wonderful family, who willingly provided invaluable back-up and support during those long hours of research and writing.

LIVE LONGER
LOOK YOUNGER

in twenty easy steps

Dr Sarah Brewer

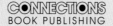

CONNECTIONS
BOOK PUBLISHING

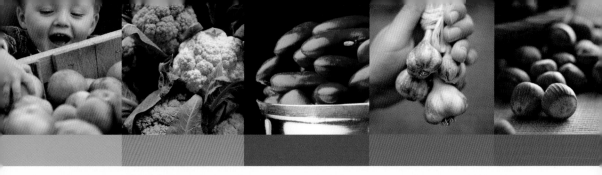

CONTENTS

BEATING AGE **6**

PART one twenty **EASY STEPS**   12

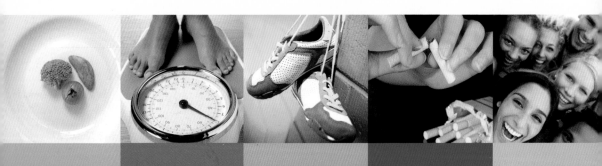

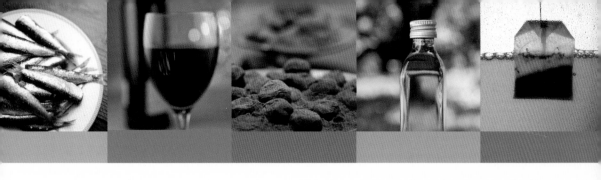

PART two body TOUR 108

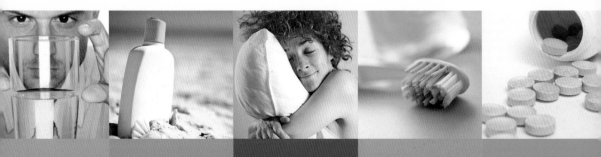

BEATING age

We can't avoid getting old – but we can certainly slow down the ageing process. Compared with just a few generations ago, when being aged fifty was considered quite old, today it merely counts as middle-aged. Average lifespans are increasing, and it's estimated that within three decades average life expectancy could be as much as 150 years. If fifty is the new forty, then 100 will become the new sixty-six within just thirty years. But we don't just want to live longer – we want to maintain our youthful vigour and extend the length of time we spend in good health, too.

Researchers have found that people who age gracefully represent a privileged group who somehow manage to avoid or overcome the illnesses to which others tend to succumb. As a result, their additional years are unusually healthy. But what about the rest of us? How can we improve our longevity and quality of life? Genes do, of course, play an important role, but don't despair – there are steps you can take to stay looking good and feeling great as you age.

Reaching the magic 100

Since the 1950s, the number of centenarians has increased faster than any other age group. Currently, an estimated one in 7,000 people reaches the age of 100, but only one in 5 million reaches the elite age of 110 to become a 'supercentenarian'. But these numbers are set to show a seven-fold increase over the next twenty-five years, so it seems we really are living longer than ever before.

And not just that. Those who reach the magic century usually stay physically younger, too: most centenarians are physically equivalent to people ten years their junior, while supercentenarians (who tend to remain physically active and independent until at least the age of 105) are equivalent to those who are twenty years younger.

The gender gap

People who live to become centenarians are more likely to have been born to a young mother aged less than twenty-five. They're also likely to be female themselves – 85 per cent of centenarians are women. Why? Possibly because they look after themselves better, drink and smoke less, and are less likely to take part in dangerous sports. Another possibility is that the oestrogen-dominant environment of the female body is more resistant to the effects of ageing. In contrast, testosterone-fuelled males are more likely to take risks, and are less likely to seek medical attention for chronic illnesses as they age. In general, men who do join the Centenarian Club tend to be those who are physically and mentally robust.

Parent power

Those with parents who live to be centenarians are more likely to live longer than those whose parents achieve only an average life expectancy. Children of centenarians also have a lower risk of developing any age-related disease – and, if these conditions do develop, they are delayed to a later age. Researchers believe this is due to a beneficial clustering of certain immune and metabolic genes: the offspring of centenarians, for example, have been found to have a type of antibody called IgM, whose characteristics more closely resemble those seen in young people rather than the elderly. Analysing this antibody might be a way of assessing someone's projected lifespan, or the effectiveness of future anti-ageing treatments.

Centenarians and supercentenarians inherit an unusually lucky combination of genes and repair systems that mean they stay healthier, for longer, as they age. They are often more resistant to the degenerative changes that contribute to ageing, and are less likely to be significantly overweight, to smoke, or to drink alcohol in excess. The combination of healthy genes and a healthy lifestyle means their extended years are spent living independently, with an agile body and mind.

So what can you do to reach your optimum age potential, and stay looking good and feeling great in the process?

Live long and prosper

Research based on a century's worth of data, collected in California since the early 1920s, suggests your personality, career trajectory and social life are at least as important to longevity as a healthy diet and exercise. The best personality predictor of longevity appears to be conscientiousness: those who are dependable rather than happy-go-lucky live the longest, whether this personality trait is assessed during childhood or in later life.

This may seem obvious, as conscientious people tend to do more things to protect their health and avoid risk-taking behaviours such as smoking, excessive drinking, drug abuse and driving too fast. They're also more likely to wear their seatbelts and follow doctor's orders. But there are other reasons, too, including genetic ones. Some people are biologically predisposed to be both more conscientious and healthier, so they are less prone to all diseases – not just those associated with dangerous habits and lifestyle. This is thought to relate to having higher levels of certain chemicals, such as serotonin, in the brain, so they are naturally less impulsive and also have better regulation of health-related habits involving appetite control and quality of sleep.

IT'S NOT TOO LATE!

Don't panic if you aren't conscientious yet – those who become so in later life (on the morning of their fortieth or fiftieth birthday, for instance!) gain enough health benefits to live longer than those who remain carefree throughout life.

And prudence isn't the only route to longevity. Researchers in the US looked at the medical histories of 424 centenarians (aged up to 119 years) to assess their resistance to ten major illnesses – high blood pressure, heart disease, diabetes, stroke, non-skin cancer, skin cancer, osteoporosis, thyroid conditions, Parkinson's disease and chronic obstructive pulmonary disease – plus cataracts. They found that centenarians formed three profiles:

- **Survivors** (24 per cent of males, 43 per cent of females) who had been diagnosed with one or more of these age-related illness before the age of eighty, but soldiered on with it.

- **Delayers** (44 per cent of males, 42 per cent of females) who did not develop any of these age-related illnesses until after the age of eighty.
- **Escapers** (32 per cent of males, 15 per cent of females) who reached the age of 100 without developing any of these common age-related illnesses.

This is good news for those of us who have lived a slightly racier life. An increasing number of centenarians are survivors who have experienced – and overcome – multiple illnesses. This suggests you don't necessarily have to have lived the life of a saint, or have a clean medical record, to reach the magical age of 100.

Other factors linked with living a long and healthy life include being a first-born child, having blood group type B, and having close relatives who've lived to at least the age of ninety-eight. Unfortunately, these factors are all beyond our control, but there are other things you can do to increase your healthy lifespan – and that's what this book is all about …

Your guide to a longer, healthier life

Did you know that flossing your teeth daily can add more than six years to your life, and eating a handful of almonds a day can lower your 'bad' cholesterol? Or that an apple a day really can keep the doctor away, while getting together with friends is actually good for your health?

In this book you'll find all the nutritional and lifestyle advice you need – based on clear scientific evidence – to help you age gracefully and stay as healthy as possible, for as long as possible. Part One reveals twenty easy ways to get started on the road to staying young and feeling great. From eating more garlic to drinking more tea, and from taking regular exercise to getting a good night's sleep, all are steps that can be easily incorporated in your day-to-day routine – there are no gruelling fitness regimes or complicated instructions to follow. You'll also find advice on the general anti-ageing supplements that are available, to help you find ones to suit your needs, if you feel that's something you might like to consider.

Part Two then goes on to take an in-depth look at different parts and functions of the body, explaining how they are most commonly affected as you age, and how you can minimize the effects of ageing through simple nutritional and lifestyle changes that provide targeted benefits to specific areas. There's also advice on useful supplements that offer anti-ageing benefits in each case.

Perhaps you've started to notice the signs of ageing and want to take action to slow down the ageing process. It's not too late – you *can* do something about it. After all, everyone wants to look and feel as young on the outside as they do on the inside – and these simple steps will show you how.

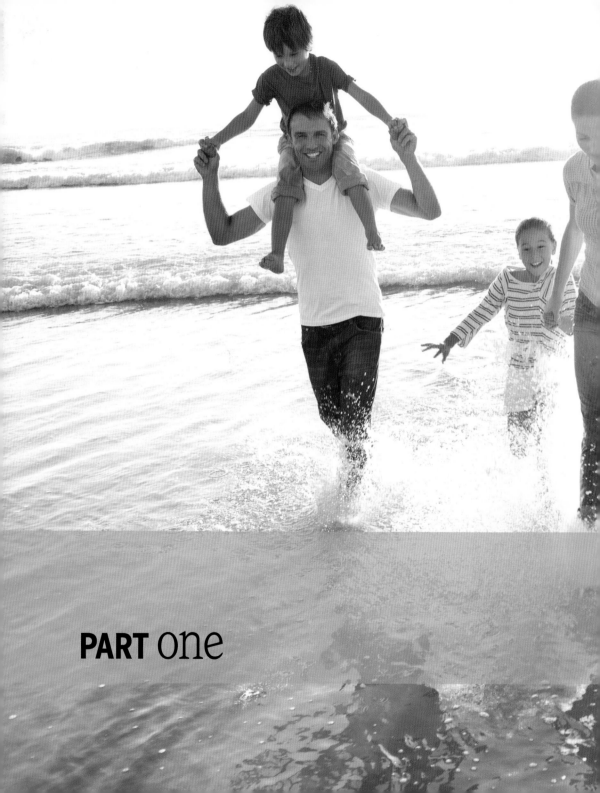

PART one

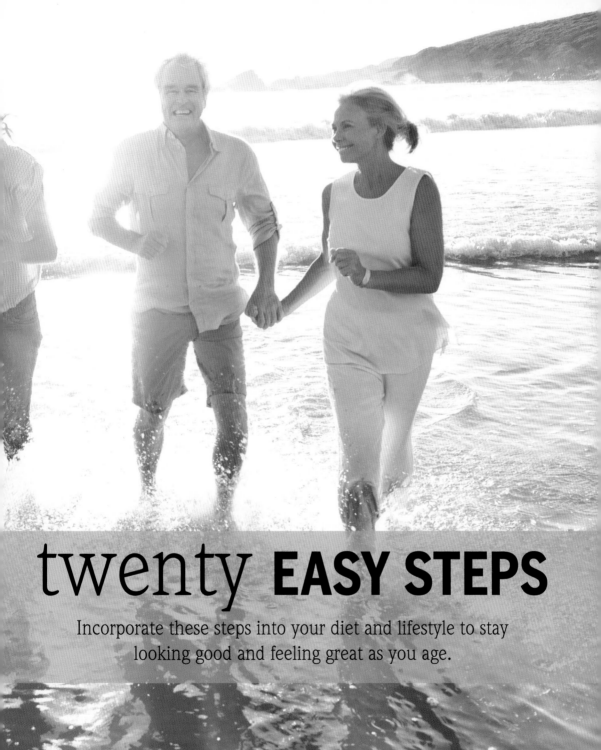

twenty **EASY STEPS**

Incorporate these steps into your diet and lifestyle to stay
looking good and feeling great as you age.

1 EAT MORE fruit

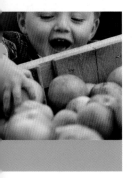

People who eat a lot of fruit tend to live longer than those who eat very little, as fruit contains a variety of beneficial substances that lower your risk of experiencing a heart attack, stroke, diabetes and many types of cancer.

Combating oxidation

Oxidation reactions are one of the leading causes of premature ageing, and a healthy diet supplying plenty of fruit (and vegetables) provides our main defence against oxidation. Oxidation reactions are triggered by chemicals known as free radicals – molecular fragments that carry a minute, negative electrical charge. This makes them highly unstable, so they try to lose the charge by passing it on (in the form of a spare electron) during collisions with other molecules and cell structures. Each of your cells undergoes an estimated 10,000 free-radical oxidations per day, which damages body proteins, fats, cell membranes and genetic material (DNA). This damage has been linked with many age-related conditions, including:

- hardening and furring-up of the arteries (atherosclerosis)
- coronary heart disease
- high blood pressure and stroke
- diabetes
- deteriorating vision due to cataracts and macular degeneration
- premature skin ageing
- chronic inflammatory diseases such as arthritis
- Alzheimer's and other forms of dementia
- Parkinson's disease
- impaired immunity
- reduced fertility
- birth defects
- cancer

FREE RADICALS

Eating fruit helps to guard against the damaging effects of free radicals. Free radicals are continuously produced in the body as a result of:

- normal (and abnormal) metabolic reactions
- muscle contraction during exercise
- smoking cigarettes
- exposure to environmental pollutants
- exposure to x-rays
- exposure to UVA sunlight
- drinking excessive amounts of alcohol
- effects of some drugs, especially antibiotics and paracetamol

Get the benefit

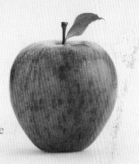

Phytochemicals, or plant substances, provide a wide range of benefits: some are powerful antioxidants, while others have beneficial hormone-like actions or anti-inflammatory effects in the body. Below are some of the phytochemicals found in fruit.

PHYTOCHEMICAL	BENEFIT
Micronutrients Vitamins, minerals and trace elements	These have essential metabolic actions needed for optimum function of all body cells. Lack of micronutrients can reduce cell activity and lead to premature ageing and cell death. Age-related increases in blood pressure are strongly related to sodium intake, and fruit contains potassium, which helps flush excess sodium from the body.
Flavonoids Red, blue, purple pigments (for example, found in red apples, black grapes, black tea and red onions)	Almost every fruit and vegetable supplies antioxidant flavonoids, of which over 20,000 are known to exist. Flavonoid antioxidants help to protect against all age-related diseases, including hardening of the arteries, diabetes and cancer.
Isoflavones Plant hormones with a weak oestrogen-like action (for example, found in soy)	These mimic the beneficial effects of oestrogen, helping to dilate coronary arteries, improve cholesterol balance and reduce blood stickiness. They improve menopausal symptoms and, by blocking stronger human oestrogens, offer some protection against cancers of the breast and prostate gland.
Phenolic and hydroxycinnamic acids (for example, found in berries, grapes and chilli peppers, as well as nuts, tea and spices)	These protect against cancer by blocking enzymes needed for growth of cancer cells.
Carotenoids Yellow, orange, red pigments (for example, found in apricots, papaya, and especially in dark green leafy vegetables)	These powerful antioxidants have beneficial effects throughout the body, including eyes, circulation and skin, and protect against cancer.

MAXIMIZE YOUR ANTIOXIDANT INTAKE

Scientists have developed a test called the Oxygen Radical Absorbance Capacity (ORAC) to assess the antioxidant potential of different foods. Originally developed by the National Institute on Aging in the US, it shows how well the antioxidants present in fruits and vegetables can mop up the harmful free radicals that contribute towards inflammation and premature ageing.

Ideally, you need to obtain at least 7,000 ORAC units per day for a good anti-ageing effect. People who consume nine servings of fruit and veg per day can obtain as many as 20,000 ORAC units from their diet alone, which significantly reduces the level of free-radical damage occurring within the body.

Take a look at the ORAC scores for various fruits listed in the table to the right, and use these to help you maximize your antioxidant intake (scores are per 100 g – equivalent to about 3½ oz).

Scientists from the University of Glasgow in the UK have also rated different fruit juices according to their antioxidant content. They found that purple grape juice, made with Concord grapes, contained the highest and broadest range of polyphenols as well as having the highest antioxidant capacity. Other high-ranking drinks include cloudy apple juice, grapefruit juice and cranberry juice drink.

FRUIT	SCORE
POMEGRANATES	10,500
CRANBERRIES	9,456
LOWBUSH BLUEBERRIES	9,260
PRUNES	8,578
PLUMS (black)	7,339
PLUMS (red)	6,239
BLACKBERRIES	5,348
RASPBERRIES	4,925
RED DELICIOUS APPLES	4,275
DATES	3,895
STRAWBERRIES	3,577
FIGS	3,383
CHERRIES	3,361
RAISINS	3,037
GALA APPLES	2,828
GOLDEN DELICIOUS APPLES	2,670
LEMONS/LIMES	2,412
PEARS (green varieties)	1,911
PEACHES	1,863
ORANGES (navel)	1,814
PEARS (Red Anjou)	1,773
TANGERINES	1,620
RED GRAPEFRUIT	1,548
RED GRAPES	1,260
GREEN GRAPES	1,118
MANGOES	1,002

Why five-a-day or more?

Guidelines throughout the world suggest eating at least five servings of fruit and vegetables per day, as researchers have found that people who eat the most fruit and vegetables have a lower risk of developing a number of chronic diseases than those who eat the least. And, while eating five a day is good, evidence suggests that eating more than five a day is considerably better! Fruit and veg help to protect against cancer, coronary heart disease, stroke and possibly diabetes, and may also reduce the risk of cataracts, diverticular disease, osteoporosis and obesity.

Cancer It's estimated that up to 70 per cent of all cancers are linked to diet. A review of over 200 clinical studies found a consistent protective effect of fruit against cancers of the stomach, oesophagus, lung, mouth/throat, uterus, pancreas and colon, so the more servings eaten, the better. One of the most protective fruits is the tomato, due to its red carotenoid pigment, lycopene (*see* page 19).

Stroke An analysis of eight studies, involving over 257,000 people, found that eating three to five servings of fruit and vegetables per day reduced the risk of stroke by 11 per cent, compared with those eating less than three a day. However, those eating more than five a day had a 26 per cent lower risk, on average. Overall, it seems that

each extra portion of fruit you eat per day reduces your risk of stroke by an additional 11 per cent.

Coronary heart disease Research involving over 278,000 people found that eating three to five servings of fruit and vegetables per day reduced the risk of coronary heart disease by 7 per cent, compared to eating fewer than three servings a day. Those who ate more than five servings per day, however, enjoyed a 17 per cent lower risk. Both fruit and vegetables provided significant protective effects against heart disease, with the greatest protection coming from citrus fruit, berries and peppers.

Diabetes A large analysis of data from ten studies involving over 190,000 people found that those with the healthiest diets (including fruit) were up to 83 per cent less likely to develop type 2 diabetes than those with a lower consumption of fruit and vegetables.

FIBRE

Fruit (and vegetables) is also an excellent source of soluble plant fibre, which helps to slow the absorption of dietary carbohydrates and fats, helping to prevent sudden rises in blood-glucose and fatty-acid levels. This is another reason why those who eat the most fruit and vegetables are the least likely to develop type 2 diabetes, coronary heart disease and stroke.

Key fruits

The following fruits are particularly beneficial. Try incorporating some of these into your diet, if possible.

- **Apricots** are a rich source of orange-yellow carotenoids. Eat a handful of dried apricots as a healthy snack two or three times a week.

DID YOU KNOW?

Eating an apple a day can reduce your risk of death from any cause, at any age, by one third. This is because apples are rich in antioxidant flavonoids that are especially protective against coronary heart disease and stroke.

- **Avocado** is a good source of vitamins C, E and betacarotene, and also contains a factor that stimulates growth of youthful skin. Aim to eat one avocado per week.

- **Cherries** contain a phytochemical called ellagic acid that protects against cancer by blocking an enzyme needed for cancer-cell growth. Eat a handful once or twice a week.

- **Chillies** contain antioxidants, such as capsaicin, that protect against coronary heart disease, cancer and premature ageing. Phytochemicals in chilli peppers thin the blood to reduce the risk of blood clots, high blood pressure and raised cholesterol levels. In some cultures, chillies are eaten every day. Try to cook with them at least once a week, if you can.

- **Citrus fruits** are an excellent source of vitamin C and bioflavonoids – powerful antioxidants that help to protect against cancer, heart disease and inflammation. Vitamin C is also vital for healthy bones and youthful skin, as it's needed to make collagen. Lemons are a rich source of limonene – a phytochemical that protects against cancer. In addition, using lime juice as a flavouring reduces the need for salt. Eat a piece of citrus fruit every day.

- **Grapes** are traditionally given during convalescence – for good reason. Red and black grapes contain antioxidants,

WHAT COUNTS AS A SERVING?

Each of these provides one serving:

- one whole apple, orange, pear, peach, nectarine, kiwi, banana, pomegranate or similar-sized fruit
- two satsumas, plums, apricots, figs, tomatoes or similar-sized fruit
- half a grapefruit, sweetie (sweet grapefruit), guava, mango, Galia melon, avocado
- a handful of grapes, cherries, blueberries, strawberries, dates
- a wine glassful (100 ml/3½ fl oz) of fruit juice (these only count towards a maximum of one serving per day, as they contain little fibre)

MIX IT UP

Choose a variety of fruit to maximize your intake of different beneficial molecules. Aim for colour on your plate – mix green, orange, yellow, red and purple fruits as much as possible. Fruit juices only count as one serving per day, however much you drink (as they have been stripped of their fibre content), but smoothies can count as two if they contain at least two full servings of whole fruit (rather than juice).

including resveratrol, that help prevent hardening and furring-up of the arteries. Grapes, like cherries, also contain ellagic acid – a phytochemical with anti-cancer properties. Eat a handful (or have a glass of red wine; *see* page 46) most days.

- **Papaya** is an excellent source of carotenoids, including the red pigment lycopene, which has anti-cancer properties. It also contains an enzyme, papain, which breaks down protein and boosts digestion. Eat it once a week.

- **Peppers** are a rich source of vitamin C, carotenoids and bioflavonoids. Weight for weight, red peppers contain three times as much vitamin C as citrus fruits (green peppers have over twice as much). Aim to eat peppers at least three times a week – add them regularly to your salads (peppers are most beneficial when eaten raw, as cooking reduces their vitamin C content).

- **Tomatoes** contain lycopene, an antioxidant red pigment that protects against coronary heart disease and some cancers, especially prostate cancer. Cooked tomatoes release their lycopene content most efficiently, so tomato ketchup and pizza sauces (surprisingly!) are among the richest dietary sources. Include tomatoes in your diet every day.

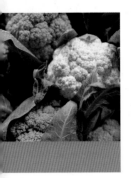

2 EAT MORE vegetables

Vegetables are a rich source of fibre, vitamins, minerals, antioxidants and plant hormones that help to protect against age-related diseases. Research consistently shows that eating more vegetables can improve your general well-being.

For every two servings of vegetables you eat, your likelihood of having a good functional health status increases, on average, by over 10 per cent. As a result, people who eat the most vegetables are more likely to live longer than those who eat the least.

Vegetables from the mustard family appear to offer the most benefit, as they are a concentrated source of substances known as glucosinolates (which impart a pungent flavour), as well as antioxidant carotenoids (yellow/orange/red plant pigments). People with the highest blood levels of carotenoids, especially one known as alpha-carotene, also appear to have an almost 40 per cent lower risk of death at any age, from any cause, including heart disease and cancer. Researchers believe this is because alpha-carotene is ten times more effective at blocking the growth of human cancer cells than similar carotenoids such as betacarotene. Alpha-carotene is found in green and yellow vegetables, especially carrots, sweet potatoes, pumpkin, butternut squash and dark green vegetables such as broccoli, green beans, spinach and lettuce.

MUSTARD FAMILY

Members of the mustard family include:

- broccoli
- cauliflower
- cabbage
- kohlrabi
- horseradish
- radish
- watercress
- kale
- bok choy (pak choi)
- Brussels sprouts
- turnip
- swede (rutabaga)

Getting enough antioxidants

The antioxidant potential of vegetables is assessed by measuring their ORAC score (for more on ORAC and the damaging effects of oxidation *see* Eat More Fruit, pages 14 and 16). The scores for different vegetables are shown opposite, to help you maximize your antioxidant intake (remember that scores are per 100 g).

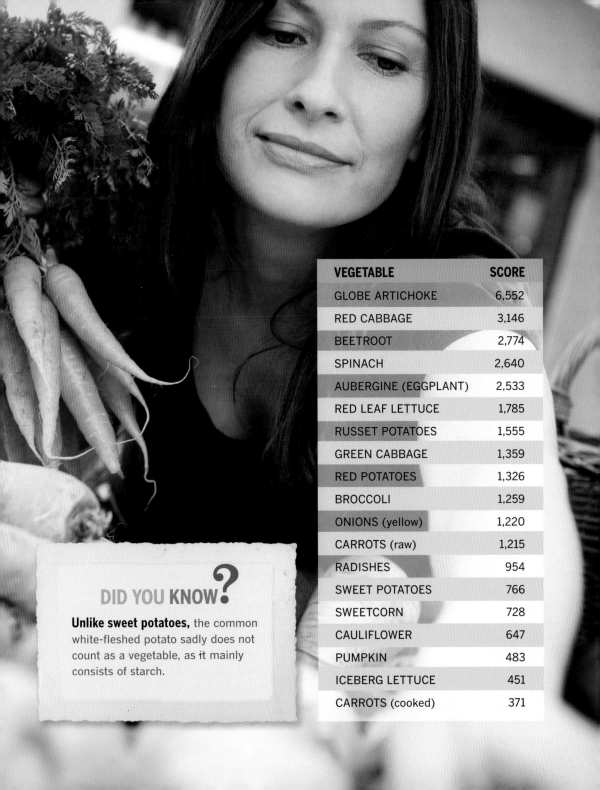

VEGETABLE	SCORE
GLOBE ARTICHOKE	6,552
RED CABBAGE	3,146
BEETROOT	2,774
SPINACH	2,640
AUBERGINE (EGGPLANT)	2,533
RED LEAF LETTUCE	1,785
RUSSET POTATOES	1,555
GREEN CABBAGE	1,359
RED POTATOES	1,326
BROCCOLI	1,259
ONIONS (yellow)	1,220
CARROTS (raw)	1,215
RADISHES	954
SWEET POTATOES	766
SWEETCORN	728
CAULIFLOWER	647
PUMPKIN	483
ICEBERG LETTUCE	451
CARROTS (cooked)	371

DID YOU KNOW?

Unlike sweet potatoes, the common white-fleshed potato sadly does not count as a vegetable, as it mainly consists of starch.

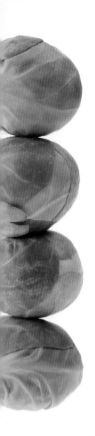

The Japanese key to longevity

The Japanese are among the longest-lived people in the world, yet there is a health gradient even across their country. Those living in Okinawa, in the south, live even longer than those in northern Japan, and have an exceptionally low risk of age-related diseases such as diabetes, heart attack, stroke and cancer. So what's their secret?

The exceptional longevity and healthy ageing of Okinawans has been attributed to their traditional, vegetable-rich diet – low in calories but supplying abundant vitamins, minerals and antioxidants. And, rather than eating rice, as in the rest of Japan, their main dietary staple is a type of sweet potato. Orange-fleshed sweet potatoes (sometimes called yams) are a rich source of carotenoids and plant hormones known as phytoestrogens. These have antioxidant actions, helping to damp down inflammation, reduce menopausal symptoms and protect against some cancers – especially those of the breast and prostate gland. Sweet potatoes are generally eaten in a similar way to normal potatoes – baked, mashed or added to vegetable soups.

Eat your greens

Elsewhere in the world, people who eat a large number of vegetables also have a lower risk of developing a number of age-related diseases; it's estimated that, in the year 2000, inadequate consumption of fruit and vegetables accounted for a staggering 2.6 million deaths worldwide. As with fruit, eating vegetables appears to offer protection against cancer, coronary heart disease, stroke and diabetes. A good vegetable intake also reduces the risk of cataracts, age-related macular degeneration (a common cause of loss of vision in later life), diverticular disease, osteoporosis and obesity.

Blood pressure Vegetables contain a number of substances that have a blood-pressure-lowering effect, including potassium, magnesium and calcium. Eating more vegetables can reduce blood pressure by around 4.0/1.5 mmHg (millimetres of mercury), which can

RECIPE FOR LIFE

A typical Okinawan meal consists of:

- miso soup, containing seaweed, tofu (soybean curd), sweet potato and green leafy vegetables
- stir-fried vegetables such as daikon radish, burdock, okra, pumpkin
- *kombu* seaweed
- *konnyaku* (a jelly-like health food made from a native sweet potato)
- small amounts of fish or boiled pork
- jasmine tea

significantly reduce your risk of a heart attack or stroke. Even in people following a healthy Mediterranean-style diet, those who eat the most vegetables are around 40 per cent less likely to have hypertension than those eating the least.

Stroke Eating three to five servings of fruit and vegetables a day reduces the risk of stroke by 11 per cent, compared to eating less than three servings a day, according to studies involving over quarter of a million people. And eating more than five servings a day lowers the risk significantly further, by 26 per cent. In addition, each extra portion of vegetables you eat a day reduces your risk by an additional 3 per cent. Eating your greens really is good for you!

Coronary heart disease Similarly, research shows that eating three to five servings of vegetables per day reduces the risk of coronary heart disease by 7 per cent, when compared to those eating fewer than three servings, while eating more than five portions a day reduces your risk by as much as 17 per cent – so, the more veg you eat, the better.

Diabetes A review of six studies involving over 223,000 people suggests that people eating the most green leafy vegetables are the least likely to develop type 2 diabetes. In fact, increasing your consumption of green leafy vegetables by one and a half portions (122 g/4¼ oz) could lower your risk of type 2 diabetes by 14 per cent.

GETTING YOUR FIVE A DAY

Aim to eat at least three (and preferably five or more) servings of different vegetables per day, excluding starchy white potatoes. Don't count (or, if possible, eat!) vegetables that are canned with salt, as their benefits are outweighed by the potentially harmful effects of sodium on your blood pressure. Aim for as much variety as possible.

Each of the following measures provides one serving:
- a handful of chopped vegetables such as carrots, cabbage, kale, sweetcorn, broccoli florets
- a small bowl of loosely packed mixed salad
- a small bowl of vegetable soup
- a wine glassful (100 ml/3½ fl oz) of vegetable juice (these only count towards a maximum of one serving per day, as they contain little fibre)

Cancer Seven out of ten cancers are linked to diet. A review of over 200 studies found that eating vegetables helps to protect against cancers of the stomach, oesophagus, lung, mouth, throat, uterus, pancreas and colon – and, the more servings you eat, the better. The greatest benefit comes from eating raw vegetables, onions, garlic, carrots, green vegetables and members of the mustard family (*see* box on page 20).

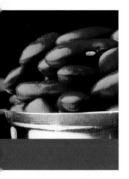

3 EAT MORE beans

Among older people, the type of food most closely associated with a longevity is – surprisingly – beans (also known as pulses or legumes). And this appears to be true regardless of where you live in the world.

Whatever your ethnic background, it seems that beans really do make you live longer. Different cultures favour different types of legume: the Japanese consume large amounts of soy, tofu, natto (fermented soybeans) and miso, for example, while Scandinavians opt for brown beans and peas and the Mediterranean diet favours lentils, chickpeas and white beans. But one fact remains constant – they're all good for you! One study involving almost 800 people aged seventy and over found that every 20 g (³/₄ oz) increase in average daily intake of beans was linked with an 8 per cent lower risk of death during the seven-year follow-up period – a protective effect that was even higher than for fish and olive oil.

LEGUMES	SCORE
RED KIDNEY BEANS	14,413
PINTO BEANS	12,359
RED LENTILS	9,766
BLACK BEANS	8,040
BLACKEYE PEAS	4,343
GREEN PEAS (fresh)	4,039
CHICKPEAS (GARBANZO)	4,030
NAVY BEANS (HARICOT)	2,474

Beating oxidation with beans

Beans are a good source of anti-ageing antioxidants. Those with the highest ORAC score are those with red or black pigments in their skin, such as red kidney beans, pinto beans, red lentils, black beans and blackeye peas (*see* left), but other types of legume, such as fresh green peas and chickpeas, score well too (for more on ORAC and the damaging effects of oxidation *see* Eat More Fruit, pages 14 and 16). Try to incorporate them in your diet whenever possible (again, scores listed are per 100 g).

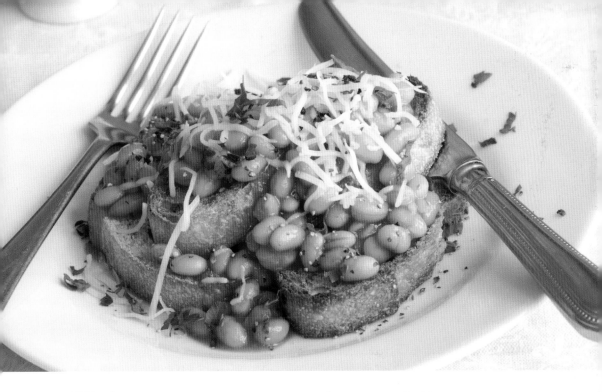

Why beans may increase longevity

Interestingly, one of the reasons beans make us live longer could actually be down to a compound they *lack* …

Dietary proteins are digested down into their basic building blocks, called amino acids. These are recycled in different types of cell to make all the proteins you need for metabolism, cell rejuvenation, tissue repair and immunity. Twenty-one amino acids are vital for human health, but nine of these can't be produced by the body and must come from our diet. These are known as the nutritionally essential amino acids.

Unlike dietary proteins of animal origin (meat, fish, eggs, dairy products), vegetable proteins (beans, nuts, seeds,

grains) do not contain all of the essential amino acids. Most beans, except soy, lack some of the essential amino acids, especially one known as methionine – and this low methionine content could explain why beans are associated with longevity: scientists have recently suggested that a restricted intake of methionine may increase lifespan, and may be as beneficial as limiting calorie intake.

In addition, although beans provide almost a fifth of their energy value in the form of carbohydrate, it is in a complex, slowly digested form which has minimal effect on blood glucose levels (in contrast to the quick energy boost, and subsequent dip, provided by simple carbohydrates, or sugars). Maintaining stable blood glucose levels

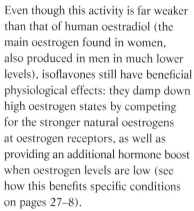

DID YOU KNOW?

On average, you need to eat around 1 g of protein per day for each kilogram (2.2 lb) of your body weight. Someone weighing 70 kg (11 st) therefore needs to obtain roughly 70 g (2½ oz) protein per day from their diet, which represents around 15 per cent of your daily energy intake.

contributes to long-term good health and can benefit appetite control, too.

How isoflavones can help

Beans, especially soy, chickpeas, lentils and mung beans, are a rich source of plant hormones known as isoflavones. Over a thousand different plant isoflavones have been identified, but only five with oestrogenic activity are found in the diet in significant amounts:

- genistein, daidzein and glycitein (mainly derived from soybeans)
- formononetin and biochanin A, which are metabolized to form daidzein and genistein (obtained mostly from chickpeas, lentils and mung beans)

As their structure is similar to that of human oestrogens, isoflavones interact with oestrogen receptors in the body.

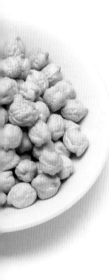

Even though this activity is far weaker than that of human oestradiol (the main oestrogen found in women, also produced in men in much lower levels), isoflavones still have beneficial physiological effects: they damp down high oestrogen states by competing for the stronger natural oestrogens at oestrogen receptors, as well as providing an additional hormone boost when oestrogen levels are low (see how this benefits specific conditions on pages 27–8).

In Japan, where soy is a dietary staple, intakes of isoflavones are 50–100 mg per day for both men and women, compared with typical Western intakes of just 2–5 mg a day – another contributing factor to the renowned longevity of the Japanese.

BENEFICIAL BACTERIA

One in three people gain even greater benefit from isoflavones, as they naturally possess sufficient numbers of probiotic intestinal bacteria (such as *Lactobacillus*, *Bacteroides*, *Bifidobacteria*) to metabolize daidzein to a more powerful oestrogen, known as equol. People can be divided into two groups: equol producers and non-equol producers. Equol has a higher antioxidant activity than other isoflavones, and equol producers therefore gain greater health benefits from isoflavones than non-equol producers. Of course, there's no way of knowing whether or not you're an equol producer, so, when eating beans or taking an isoflavone supplement, it's therefore also worth taking a probiotic supplement supplying these beneficial digestive bacteria.

Menopausal symptoms In Japan, where isoflavone intake is high, less than 25 per cent of women experience hot flushes at the menopause, compared with 85 per cent of Western women. A number of studies suggest that isoflavones can reduce menopausal symptoms such as hot flushes and night sweats, while a recent analysis of nineteen clinical trials found that isoflavones significantly reduced hot flushes by 39 per cent, compared with placebo.

Heart disease Isoflavones can reduce the risk of coronary heart disease in a variety of ways, including through their antioxidant and anti-inflammatory actions, which protect against hardening and furring-up of the arteries. By interacting with oestrogen receptors, isoflavones promote dilation of coronary arteries, reduce arterial stiffness, reduce abnormal blood-clotting and have a blood-pressure-lowering effect. They also have beneficial effects on cholesterol balance. Although much of this

research involved post-menopausal women, isoflavones have also been shown to reduce the risk of coronary heart disease among high-risk, middle-aged males.

Bone health Isoflavones mimic the effects of natural oestrogen on bones and may help to protect against osteoporosis. Studies show that post-menopausal women with high intakes of dietary isoflavones have significantly greater bone-mineral density, at both their spine and hip, than those with the lowest intakes, even after adjusting for age, height, weight, years since menopause, smoking, alcohol consumption, HRT usage and daily calcium intake. The protective effects of soy isoflavones in maintaining bone-mineral density appear to be most marked in women in later menopause,

Fresh peas are a good source of antioxidants.

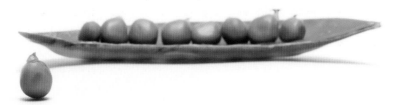

and in those with a lower body weight or lower calcium intake.

Hormone-sensitive cancers

Isoflavones may play an important role in protecting against hormone-sensitive cancers such as those of the breast and prostate gland. By blocking oestrogen receptors to reduce overall stimulation from stronger human oestrogens, they help to protect hormone-sensitive tissues. Research involving over 21,000 Japanese women and 35,000 Singapore Chinese women suggests that those with the highest intake of soy isoflavones are half as likely to develop breast cancer as those with the lowest intake – even after adjusting for factors such as reproductive history, family history, smoking, other dietary considerations and weight. The protection was highest in post-menopausal women. Studies in Japan and Korea also suggest that men who are equol producers have a lower incidence of prostate cancer than non-equol producers, and that a diet based on soybean isoflavones is useful in preventing prostate cancer.

Memory A diet rich in soy isoflavones has been found to improve memory and frontal-lobe function in young healthy students (both male and female), in men awaiting gender reassignment and in postmenopausal women. The greatest improvements are seen in memory recall, sustained-attention tasks, planning tasks, verbal memory and learning rule reversals.

Bring on the beans!

Eat beans regularly by adding them to salads, soups, stir-fries, stews and casseroles. All have a low glycemic index (for more information on a low-GI diet *see* Part Two, page 128).

● **Chickpeas** are good source of protein but, as with many pulses, some important amino acids are missing. They are therefore best combined with other plant foods and wholegrains such as rice and bread to provide a balanced amino-acid intake. Chickpeas are a good source of potassium, calcium, magnesium and folate, and also contain useful amounts of iron, zinc, manganese, selenium, vitamin E and B group vitamins. As well as using them in soups and stews, why not try making hummus – the popular Middle Eastern dish which combines mashed chickpeas with lemon juice, olive oil and tahini (sesame paste).

● **Soybeans** contain all the essential amino acids and are therefore considered of comparable nutritional quality to meats. They are also a good source of calcium, potassium, magnesium, iron, zinc, manganese, B group vitamins, folate and selenium. Soybeans are available in red-, black- and white-coloured varieties, and are now added to many functional foods such as muesli bars and bread for their immense health benefits. Add to soups, stews and casseroles, eat young 'twig' beans boiled or steamed as a healthy

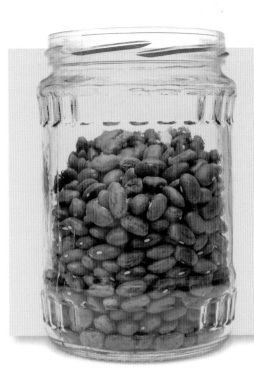

Dried kidney beans should be boiled rapidly for at least 15 minutes, then simmered until thoroughly cooked. This denatures substances (lectins) which can otherwise lead to indigestion and symptoms similar to food poisoning (which, unbelievably, can occur when as few as five incorrectly prepared beans are eaten!). Soaking beans overnight reduces cooking times, and also helps to deactivate the indigestible sugars that are fermented by bacteria to produce intestinal wind.

snack (edamame), or use soy products such as tofu, miso, soy milk and soy sauce. Soybeans are such a rich source of isoflavones that as little as 60 g (2 oz) per day (supplying around 45 mg isoflavones) can provide significant, anti-ageing benefits.

● **Lentils** are available in numerous varieties such as yellow, red, green, gold and brown. They are a good source of oestrogenic substances, including isoflavones and lignans (another phytochemical). They are ideal for adding to soups, stews, casseroles, flans and rissoles, and are widely used in Asia to make dhal, which, when served with rice, helps to provide a balanced intake of amino acids. Lentils also contain useful amounts of potassium,

magnesium, iron, copper, zinc, selenium and B group vitamins. Red lentils also provide a small amounts of carotenoid pigments.

● **Kidney beans** are available in red, white or black varieties, with the darkest types supplying the highest level of antioxidants. They are an excellent source of protein, and are a staple part of the diet in many parts of the world, especially Central and South America. To balance their lack of certain amino acids, they are best eaten in a combination of five parts rice to one part beans. Kidney beans provide twice as much fibre as green beans, are a good source of potassium, and also contain useful amounts of folate, calcium, magnesium, iron, zinc and selenium.

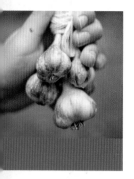

4 EAT MORE garlic

Garlic is such a popular culinary herb that, worldwide, average consumption is equivalent to one clove per person per day. And the good news for garlic lovers is that it just happens to be an anti-ageing superfood.

Garlic (*Allium sativum*) is more than just a delicious seasoning; it has an astonishing range of health-giving properties, too. According to studies on the beneficial effects of garlic (based on consuming 600–900 mg dried garlic tablets – equivalent to 1.8–2.7 g fresh garlic – per day), garlic boasts the following array of benefits:

- antioxidant
- anti-inflammatory
- anti-bacterial
- anti-viral
- anti-cancer
- blood-thinning
- cholesterol lowering
- blood-pressure lowering
- homocysteine (an amino acid) lowering

And, if you need any further convincing of its value, read on …

Garlic power

The antioxidant ORAC score of raw garlic is surprisingly low (*see* table on page 33), but this is because most of the antioxidant potential is 'locked up'

in the form of an odourless substance called alliin. When garlic is cut or crushed, alliin is released from damaged cells to interact with a garlic enzyme, to release a unique substance called allicin. Allicin is what gives crushed garlic its characteristic smell.

Allicin and sulphur compounds formed by its breakdown in aged garlic are powerful antioxidants. When consumed, they are rapidly absorbed into the body to protect circulating 'bad' LDL (low-density lipoprotein) cholesterol from oxidation. As a result, unoxidized LDL-cholesterol is not attacked and absorbed by scavenger cells and taken in to artery walls but, instead, is taken up by 'good' HDL (high-density lipoprotein) cholesterol, which transports it back to the liver for processing. In this way, regular garlic consumption helps to protect against hardening and furring-up of the arteries (atherosclerosis).

Cholesterol As well as reducing cholesterol oxidation, allicin prevents cells from taking up cholesterol, reduces cholesterol production in the liver and

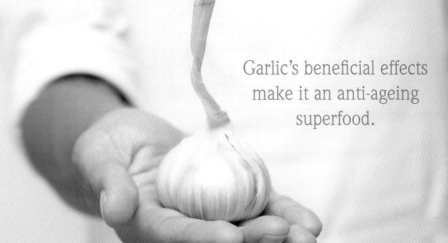

Garlic's beneficial effects make it an anti-ageing superfood.

promotes the excretion of fatty acids to further discourage atherosclerosis. Researchers have found that daily consumption of garlic reduces total cholesterol levels by around 10 per cent.

Blood pressure Garlic extracts can lower a raised blood pressure by an average of 16.3/9.3 mmHg – enough to reduce the risk of a stroke by up to 40 per cent. Interestingly, it doesn't seem to reduce a normal blood pressure in people without an elevated systolic blood pressure (the amount of pressure blood exerts on vessels while the heart is beating). The effect is a gradual process, occurring with a minimum of two to three months of consuming garlic regularly, and is thought to result from decreased blood stickiness,

HOMOCYSTEINE AND HEALTH

When homocysteine builds up in the circulation, it damages the lining of artery walls so they become narrow and inelastic. Some research suggests that a raised homocysteine level is as important a risk factor for heart disease as a raised cholesterol level. It's also associated with other ageing conditions, including Alzheimer's disease. Homocysteine levels are commonly lowered by folic acid, vitamin B_{12} and vitamin B_6.

changes in the way salts move in and out of cells, and by relaxing the smooth muscle lining of artery walls.

Homocysteine Elevated blood levels of the amino acid homocysteine, naturally produced in the body, are

GETTING THE MOST FROM YOUR GARLIC

If garlic is cooked immediately after cutting or crushing, the production of allicin is inactivated, and some anti-ageing benefits are lost. So – at the risk of losing some friends! – garlic is best consumed raw or in the form of enteric-coated capsules for maximum effect. As the amount of allicin in garlic varies considerably depending on where and how it's grown, it's best to take standardized garlic-powder tablets, which provide a guaranteed dose of allicin. Enteric coating reduces garlic odour on breath and protects the active ingredients from degradation in the stomach.

of cell cycles (in other words, a direct slowing of cell ageing) and by reducing the formation of harmful chemicals (nitrosamines) within the body. A daily intake of 5 g garlic (two to three cloves) appears to completely block nitrosamine production.

Viral infections Taking garlic regularly also appears to reduce the risk of developing a cold. Although not specifically related to ageing, this does suggest a boost in immunity, which may well be associated with anti-ageing benefits. In a study in which just under 150 people were given either garlic supplements or inactive placebo for twelve weeks, only twenty-four of those on garlic developed a cold, compared with sixty-five of those taking dummy tablets. Those taking garlic also had shorter colds, lasting for one and a half days less than for those not taking garlic.

Garlic also has other beneficial effects, including lowering blood levels of triglycerides (a harmful type of blood fat), reducing abnormal blood-clotting and improving blood fluidity. And, by dilating small arteries (arterioles) and small veins (venules), garlic also improves blood flow to the skin by almost 50 per cent, which can enhance youthful glow and supply more oxygen and nutrients to slow skin ageing. This blood-vessel-dilation effect can be measured in nail-bed folds within as few as 5 hours of taking just a single dose.

linked with hardening and furring-up of the arteries. Garlic extracts have recently been shown to help lower homocysteine levels – a beneficial effect that is under further investigation.

Coronary heart disease Regular consumption of garlic – thanks to its wealth of beneficial effects – is believed to lower the risk of a heart attack and premature death by as much as 50 per cent in men and 30 per cent in women.

Cancer Garlic is thought to reduce the risk of cancer through its direct, protective effect on genetic material (DNA) in cells, which reduces mutations, by slowing the progression

WELL-BEING WONDER

Garlic doesn't just provide physical health benefits – it can boost our general well-being, too. A study assessing psychological state before and after taking garlic daily for four months found that those taking garlic extracts experienced a marked improvement in positive mood characteristics (activity, elated mood, concentration, sensitivity) and a drop in negative mood characteristics (anxiety, irritation), while those taking inactive placebo noticed no significant mood changes.

Other anti-ageing herbs and spices

A number of other culinary herbs and spices have a surprisingly high antioxidant ORAC score (*see* Eat More Fruit, page 16), even though you only eat them in small amounts. The table to the right lists ORAC values per gram – not per 100 g, as for fruit and vegetables. Adding just 1 g of black pepper to a meal gives you an additional 301 ORAC units, while a single gram of cinnamon supplies an amazing 2,675 ORAC units – so start spicing up your meals!

SPICE/HERB	SCORE
CLOVES	3,144
CINNAMON	2,675
OREGANO	2,001
TURMERIC	1,592
NUTMEG	1,572
CUMIN	768
PARSLEY	743
BASIL LEAF	676
SAFFRON	530
CURRY POWDER	485
SAGE LEAF	320
BLACK PEPPERCORNS	301
MUSTARD SEED	292
GINGER POWDER	288
THYME	274
CHILLI POWDER	236
PAPRIKA	179
MINT	139
GARLIC	54

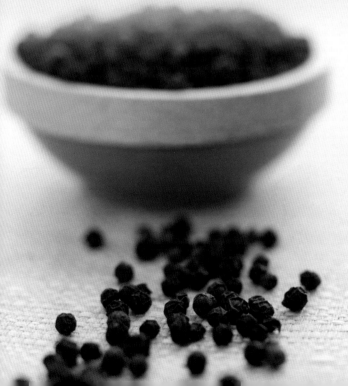

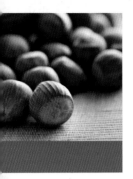

5 EAT MORE nuts

Nuts are an important weapon in your anti-ageing arsenal. The edible kernels are a rich source of antioxidants, vitamins, minerals and essential oils that protect against a variety of age-related conditions.

People who eat a high quantity of nuts – 'nature's own perfect health food' – tend to have a significantly lower risk of developing high blood pressure, raised cholesterol levels, type 2 diabetes, coronary heart disease and stroke. Research also suggests that they live two to three years longer than those who eat hardly any nuts at all.

Nuts are an excellent source of fibre, which helps to slow the absorption of dietary sugars and cholesterol, and they have a high protein content, averaging around 20 per cent. In addition, nut protein has a filling effect, helping to curb appetite.

Nuts are also a rich source of antioxidants (*see* table opposite), including plant hormones known as phytoestrogens. These have a weak, oestrogen-like effect in the body that helps to protect against many age-related conditions, including breast cancer in women and prostate cancer in men. They can also reduce menopausal symptoms such as hot flushes by up to 40 per cent.

Going nuts

Try adding nuts to cereals, muesli, salads, yogurts and desserts. Have a handful (30–60 g/1–2 oz) of mixed, unsalted nuts every day, as a healthy snack. Buy them fresh, little and often, for maximum freshness, from a shop with a rapid turnover. Use nut oils in salad dressings for a delicious

DID YOU KNOW?

Brazil nuts are the richest dietary source of selenium – a mineral that can halve your risk of developing cancer.

Walnuts are a good source of omega-3 essential fatty acids that help to protect against heart disease.

Macadamia nuts and hazelnuts are a rich source of beneficial monounsaturated fatty acids – the same type found in olive oil.

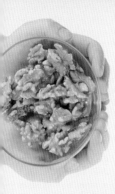

Supernuts

The ten supernuts below are among the most popular and useful for beating age. ORAC scores listed are per 100 g – use the scores to maximize your antioxidant intake. You can get 20,000 ORAC units (the magic number for optimum protection) just from eating a bag of pecan nuts! (For more on ORAC and the effects of oxidation *see* Eat More Fruit, pages 14 and 16.)

NUT	SCORE	OTHER NUTRITIONAL BENEFITS
PECAN NUTS	17,940	Good source of monounsaturated fats, potassium, zinc, manganese and vitamin E.
WALNUTS	13,541	Rich source of omega-3 essential oils, vitamin E and selenium.
HAZELNUTS	9,645	Excellent source of vitamin E, and a good source of potassium, iron, manganese and monounsaturated fats such as oleic acid.
PISTACHIOS	7,983	Excellent source of potassium, vitamin E and carotenoid antioxidants (in the green lining).
ALMONDS	4,454	Excellent source of vitamin E, and a good source of potassium, calcium and zinc.
PEANUTS	3,166	Good source of magnesium, manganese, zinc and vitamins E, B3 and biotin.
CASHEWS	1,948	Lower fat content than most nuts, but most is in the form of beneficial monounsaturated fats. Good source of potassium, magnesium, iron, manganese and zinc.
MACADAMIAS	1,695	One of the best dietary sources of monounsaturated fats such as oleic acid, and a good source of vitamin E and selenium.
BRAZIL NUTS	1,419	The richest dietary source of selenium, and a good source of potassium, magnesium, calcium and zinc.
PINE NUTS	720	Good source of potassium, iron, magnesium, manganese and zinc, and an excellent source of vitamin E. Most of its fats are polyunsaturated and monounsaturated.

alternative to regular vinaigrette. Nut milks make a refreshing drink that is lactose, dairy and soy free – useful for those with a cow's milk intolerance. Nut milks are widely available in health-food stores, but you can easily make your own – you just need some nuts and water (*see* recipe below). Nuts also have a low glycemic index (for more information on a low-GI diet *see* Part Two, pages 128–9).

MAKE YOUR OWN NUT MILK
You will need:
45 g (1½ oz) raw almonds, cashews or macadamia nuts
200 ml (6¾ fl oz) filtered or mineral water

- Soak the nuts in water overnight.
- Place all ingredients in a blender. Pulse a few times to break up the nuts and then blend at high speed for at least a minute, until the nuts are completely broken down.
- Strain the liquid through a fine wire-mesh strainer or muslin cloth, using a spoon or spatula to help push the milk through.
- Cover and refrigerate. The milk will keep in the refrigerator for two days.

Try adding honey, vanilla extract, cinnamon or cocoa for a range of delicious flavours.

- **Almonds** Eating a handful of almonds a day (about twenty-three kernels) can lower your 'bad' LDL-cholesterol by 5 per cent and increase your 'good' HDL-cholesterol by 6 per cent. This can improve your cholesterol balance enough to reduce your risk of a heart attack or stroke by as much as 20 per cent. Almond oil offers similar cholesterol-lowering benefits.

- **Brazil nuts** are the richest dietary source of selenium – a mineral that is arguably the most important trace element in our diet. Selenium provides protection against a number of age-related health problems, and is essential for a healthy immune system. It increases the activity of scavenger white blood cells, and is involved in the production of antibodies which help to reduce the severity of viral illnesses. It also plays a vital role in lowering the risk of cancer. And the good news is that you can meet your optimum selenium intake by eating just two or three Brazil nuts a day.

- **Cashew nuts** are unusual in that the nut hangs from the cashew 'fruit' (which is really a swollen stalk) rather than being encased by it. In Brazil, cashew nuts are considered to have a rejuvenating, aphrodisiac action, in addition to their nutritional benefits.

- **Hazelnuts** are a rich source of monounsaturated fatty acids, with hazelnut oil containing as much as

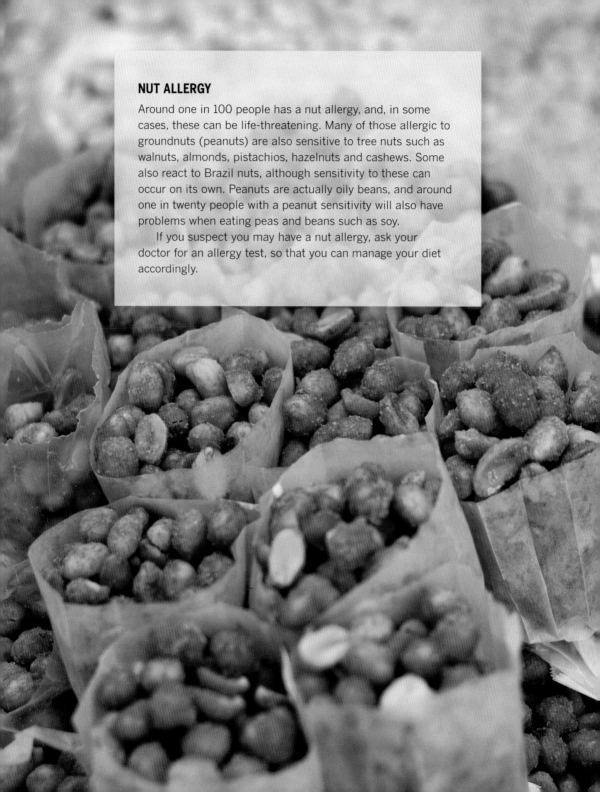

NUT ALLERGY

Around one in 100 people has a nut allergy, and, in some cases, these can be life-threatening. Many of those allergic to groundnuts (peanuts) are also sensitive to tree nuts such as walnuts, almonds, pistachios, hazelnuts and cashews. Some also react to Brazil nuts, although sensitivity to these can occur on its own. Peanuts are actually oily beans, and around one in twenty people with a peanut sensitivity will also have problems when eating peas and beans such as soy.

If you suspect you may have a nut allergy, ask your doctor for an allergy test, so that you can manage your diet accordingly.

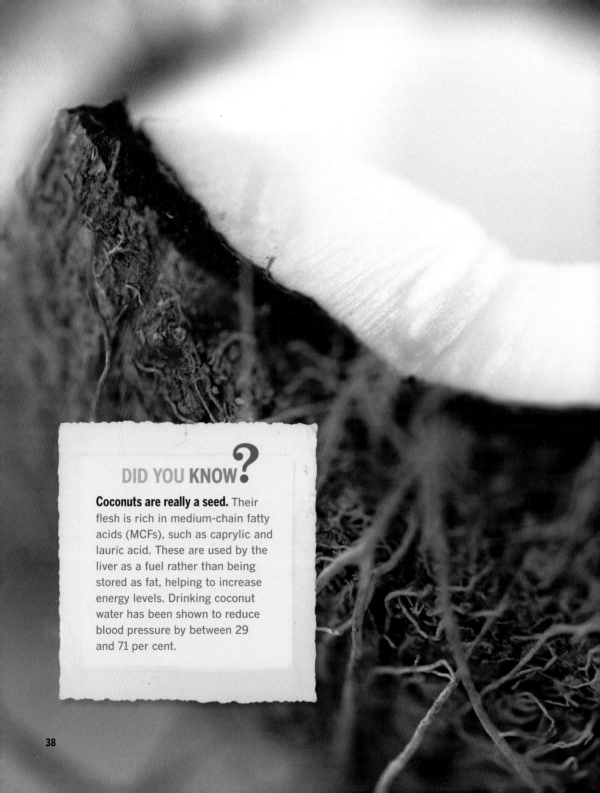

DID YOU KNOW?

Coconuts are really a seed. Their flesh is rich in medium-chain fatty acids (MCFs), such as caprylic and lauric acid. These are used by the liver as a fuel rather than being stored as fat, helping to increase energy levels. Drinking coconut water has been shown to reduce blood pressure by between 29 and 71 per cent.

82 per cent – higher than for olive oil (73 per cent) and almond oil (68 per cent), and similar to that of macadamia nut oil (81 per cent). Eating a serving of hazelnuts every day significantly raises blood levels of vitamin E and lowers total cholesterol and harmful LDL-cholesterol.

● **Macadamias,** along with hazelnuts, are one of the richest dietary sources of monounsaturated fatty acids, containing 81 per cent. Eating a diet enriched with macadamia nuts has been shown to significantly lower both total blood cholesterol and LDL-cholesterol within three weeks. These effects were seen when eating as little as 20 g (³/₄ oz) of macadamias a day. Slight reductions in weight and BMI (body mass index – *see* page 67) also occurred, despite an increase in the total amount of fat consumed, as macadamias contain protein and fibre that help to fill you up and curb your appetite.

● **Peanuts, or groundnuts,** are not tree nuts but legumes – like beans. They are a good source of resveratrol – an antioxidant also found in red wine. Resveratrol is believed to protect against hardening and furring-up of the arteries (atherosclerosis) and coronary heart disease.

● **Pistachios** help to lower 'bad' LDL-cholesterol and increase 'good' HDL-cholesterol to reduce furring-up of the arteries and the risk of heart attack. They may also help to protect against diabetes, due to their high content of beneficial monounsaturated and essential fatty acids. Like macadamias, pistachios help to fill you up and curb appetite, so, even though they are nutrient-dense and contain significant calories, they help you maintain a healthy weight.

● **Walnuts** are a rich source of omega-3 essential oils that, like fish oils, have a beneficial effect on cholesterol balance as well as reducing inflammation. Regular consumption of walnuts can lower 'bad' LDL-cholesterol enough to reduce the risk of coronary heart disease by 30–50 per cent and add an estimated five to ten years to your life.

Macadamias and pistachios help fill you up, so can be useful when you're trying to maintain a healthy weight.

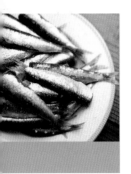

6 EAT MORE oily fish

The omega-3 fatty acids found in oily fish provide exceptional anti-ageing benefits for virtually all parts of the body, including heart, joints and brain. It's therefore vital to ensure you're getting enough in your diet.

As we evolved from the sea, it's not surprising that fish features prominently in some of the healthiest diets in the world. Those following Mediterranean-, Eskimo- and Japanese-style diets have an unusually low risk of developing high blood pressure, coronary heart disease, stroke, diabetes and even depression. These protective effects of fish are due to the beneficial oils they contain.

Omega-3 and omega-6

There are two main types of polyunsaturated fatty acids: omega-3s and omega-6s. Their names derive from their chemical structure, which determines how they are processed by the body.

- **Omega-3s**, which are mainly found in oily fish, are converted into a series of hormone-like substances that have powerful anti-ageing, anti-inflammatory effects in the body.
- **Omega-6s** (mainly derived from vegetable oils), in contrast, are mostly converted into substances that *promote* inflammation.

Our traditional, Stone Age, hunter-gatherer diet of green plants, wild animals and fish provided equal amounts of omega-6s (from natural vegetable oils) and omega-3s (from oily fish). But most people following a Western diet now obtain at least seven times more omega-6s (from margarines, spreads, processed and ready meals) than omega-3s, which increases the risk of ageing inflammatory conditions, including coronary heart disease and stroke.

How fish oils help

Scientists have calculated that, for every 20 g ($^3/_4$ oz) increase in fish and shellfish you eat, you enjoy a 6 per cent lower chance of dying, at any age, from any medical cause, even after taking smoking into account.

Diabetes Research shows that older people who eat the most fish are 60 per cent less likely to develop poor glucose control and diabetes than those who eat no fish, even when factors such as age, weight and carbohydrate are considered.

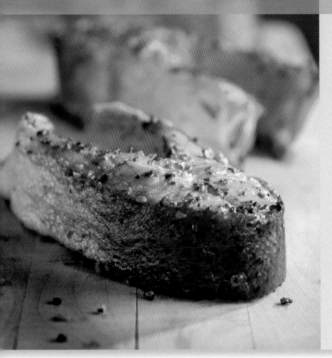

Fresh salmon is a rich source of beneficial omega-3s.

OILY FISH

Your body cannot convert omega-6 fatty acids into omega-3s, so a good supply of dietary omega-3s is vital. Fish classed as oily include:

Anchovies (unsalted) • Bloater • Cacha • Carp • Eel • Herring • Hilsa • Jack fish • Katla • Kipper • Mackerel • Orange roughy • Pangas • Pilchards • Salmon • Sardines • Sprats • Swordfish • Trout • Tuna (fresh, but not tinned) • Whitebait

Non-fish sources of omega-3s include blue-green algae, walnuts, flax seed and hempseed oils.

Heart disease Even a modest increase in dietary intake of oily fish can help to prevent death due to coronary thrombosis (heart attack). In those who have already had a heart attack, eating more fish significantly reduces the likelihood of having a second attack – and, if one does occur, the chance of dying from it is significantly decreased. Fish oils reduce blood stickiness, abnormal blood-clotting and abnormal heart rhythms, and also have a beneficial effect on the level of triglyceride fats in the blood. Some research suggests that fish oils also improve the elasticity of artery walls.

The protective effects of consuming fish oils develop within just four weeks of increasing consumption. This rapid effect is thought to result from a thinning effect on the blood, which reduces the chance of blood clots. Benefits continue so that, after two years, those on a high-fish diet are almost a third less likely to die from a heart attack than those eating little fish. Interestingly, however, overall, omega-3s appear to have a neutral effect on cholesterol balance (or may slightly raise 'good' HDL-cholesterol and slightly lower 'bad' LDL-cholesterol, with no change in total cholesterol), although this depends on the genes you've inherited.

Stroke A large analysis of data from six studies suggests that eating any fish on a weekly basis reduces the risk of stroke by 12 per cent, with possible additional reductions of 2 per cent per serving per week. Other studies agree that eating oily fish two to four times a week can lower your risk of a stroke by over a quarter, while eating fish five or more times a week can reduce the risk of a stroke by more than a half.

Inflammatory disease Eating fish two or three times a week has been shown to reduce the risk of inflammatory bowel disease, rheumatoid arthritis and psoriasis. People who eat oily fish at least twice a week are also half as likely to experience asthma, wheezing or chest tightness on waking, compared to those who eat little oily fish – even when factors such as smoking are taken into account. Fish oils also reduce the severity of exercise-induced asthma by damping down inflammation in the airways.

Osteoarthritis Increasing intakes of omega-3 fish oils reduces the level of inflammatory chemicals within arthritic joints that are responsible for increased blood flow, heat and pain. Omega-3s appear to have a pain-killing action similar to that of non-steroidal anti-inflammatory drugs, and can reduce the amount of analgesics you need to take.

Brain health Fatty acids found in oily fish are involved in communication between brain cells and play important structural roles within brain-cell membranes, improving their fluidity so that messages are passed on more rapidly from one cell to another. A good intake of oily fish or fish oil supplements can reduce the risk of depression, improve memory and may help to protect against age-related cognitive decline and dementia.

Cancer Fish oils may have a role in reducing the risk of cancer, by interfering with the growth of tumour cells and reversing the weight loss that can occur in people with cancer. A number of trials suggest that each additional 100 g (3½ oz) of fish you consume per week lowers the risk of bowel cancer by around 3 per cent.

Improving your omega balance

Fish oils have such a powerful, beneficial effect on health that some experts recommend you eat at least 300 g of oily fish (10½ oz) per week. For most people, this means increasing your average fish intake by a factor of ten! To improve your omega balance:

Consume more omega-3s, found in:
- oily fish (two to four portions a week)
- wild-game meat such as venison and buffalo

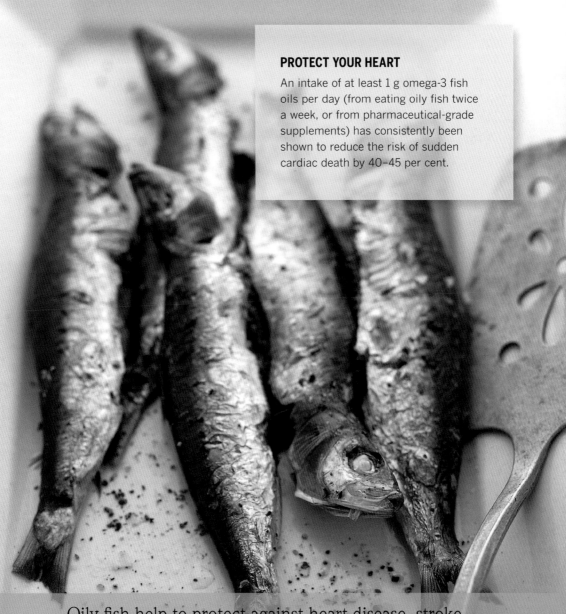

PROTECT YOUR HEART

An intake of at least 1 g omega-3 fish oils per day (from eating oily fish twice a week, or from pharmaceutical-grade supplements) has consistently been shown to reduce the risk of sudden cardiac death by 40–45 per cent.

Oily fish help to protect against heart disease, stroke, osteoarthritis and even depression.

- grass-fed beef
- omega-3-enriched eggs
- walnuts and walnut oil
- omega-3 fish oil supplements

Cut out excess omega-6s by comsuing less:
- omega-6 vegetable oils such as safflower oil, sunflower oil, grape seed oil, corn oil, cottonseed oil or soybean oil
- margarines based on omega-6 oils, such as sunflower or safflower oil
- convenience foods
- fast foods
- manufactured goods such as cakes, sweets and pastries

MAKE SURE IT'S FRESH

Fresh fish should smell of seawater – salty, with a tang of ozone and slightly sweet. It should *not* smell of fish. This characteristic smell comes from the breakdown of chemicals – so, if your fish smells fishy, it's a sure sign that it's not as fresh as possible.

Fresh fish skin should gleam like expensive shot silk and feel young and firm to the touch: when you push a finger into the flesh, it should spring back with elasticity and not remain collapsed and dented. Scales (if any) should be tight rather than loose, and, on cutting, the flesh should feel firm and tight, not flabby, waterlogged or flaky. Inspect the eyes of fish you are buying, as those of fresh produce are clear, bright, shiny and gleaming; once the fish starts to deteriorate, the eyes become shrunken and cloudy. Also, check the gills of your potential purchase, which should be a healthy pink or bright red – not a dingy brown.

When fish is guaranteed absolutely ultra-fresh, it is delicious and exceptionally good for health when eaten raw, Japanese style (as Sushi or Sashimi), for the greatest anti-ageing benefits.

FISH OIL SUPPLEMENTS

Many people don't like preparing or eating fish. To ensure you obtain the protective anti-ageing benefits of omega-3s, a fish oil supplement therefore becomes essential. The dose you need depends on your diet, and the amount of oily fish you normally tend to eat.

For general health in younger adults, a minimum intake of 450 mg long-chain omega-3 fish oils (DHA and EPA) is needed per day. To reduce the risk of heart disease, those aged fifty and over should consider taking 1 g omega-3 fish oils to help protect against heart attack, and for beneficial effects on joints and brain health. For those with significant joint pain and swelling (arthritis),

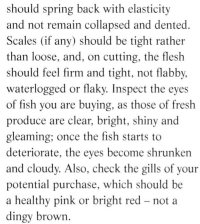

higher intakes of 3–6 g omega-3 fish oils per day may be needed for a good anti-inflammatory effect.

HOW MUCH DO YOU GET FROM YOUR DIET?

The average adult following a Western-style diet eats just 50 g (1¼ oz) of oily fish a week, supplying a meagre 1 g of the beneficial long-chain omega-3s (EPA/DHA). An extraordinary 70 per cent of adults eat no oily fish at all. The table below shows how many of the beneficial long-chain omega-3s are found in a typical portion of different types of fish.

If you eat little or no oily fish, then your anti-ageing fish oil supplement

needs to provide at least 450 mg EPA/DHA per day for general health, 1 g per day for heart-health benefits and 3 g or more per day if your painful joints have not responded to a lower dose. Invest in a super-strength or premium product.

FISH	PORTION SIZE (grams)	LONG-CHAIN OMEGA-3s per portion	
KIPPERS	150 g	3.89 g	EXCELLENT
SALMON	150 g	3.25 g	
MACKEREL	150 g	2.89 g	
PILCHARDS (in tomato sauce)	110 g	2.86 g	
HERRING	150 g	1.97 g	GOOD
TUNA (fresh)	150 g	1.95 g	
TROUT	150 g	1.73 g	
SARDINES in tomato sauce	100 g	1.67 g	
TINNED SALMON (in brine, drained)	100 g	1.55 g	
PLAICE	150 g	0.45 g	POOR
COD	150 g	0.38 g	
HADDOCK	150 g	0.24 g	
TINNED TUNA (in oil, drained)	45 g	0.17 g	
TINNED TUNA (in brine, drained)	45 g	0.08 g	

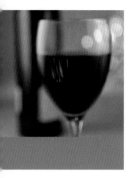

7 ENJOY A GLASS OF
red wine

You may be surprised to learn that drinking a small glass of red wine a day is actually good for you! This is thanks to the wide variety of antioxidants it contains, which do wonders for our heart health.

Interest in the anti-ageing benefits of red wine initially arose because of the so-called French Paradox. French researchers noted (with some satisfaction) that, compared with Brits and Americans, the French ate as much saturated fat, had similar high cholesterol levels, smoked as much (if not more), and did just as little exercise, yet their risk of heart disease was lower than for any other industrialized country except Japan (the Japanese, of course, being protected by their high intake of omega-3 fish oils and soy isoflavones).

This paradox was most evident in Gascony – home of the fatty Toulouse sausage and the cardiologist's ultimate nightmare, pâté de foie gras.

The main difference identified between these nations' dietary habits was intake of wine, which the French usually enjoyed alongside their food. One study found that, within seventeen countries where wine consumption was known, wine was the only 'foodstuff' with a significant protective effect against age-related mortality in adults. So what's the key?

The magic ingredients

Wine is a complex liquid, containing a wide variety of antioxidants such as flavonoids, flavonols, catechins, soluble tannins, anthocyanins and procyanidins. Wine also contains natural anti-fungal agents, such as resveratrol, found in the skins of grapes. Because grape juice is left in contact with grape skins for longer during red wine production, it contains significantly higher concentrations of these powerful antioxidants than white wine or champagne.

A HEARTY DRINK

A large analysis of data from thirty-four studies, involving over a million people, showed that risk of coronary heart disease decreased with intakes of up to four drinks per day in men, and up to two drinks in women. Overall, research suggests that drinking up to 150 ml (5 fl oz) wine per day is likely to do more good than harm.

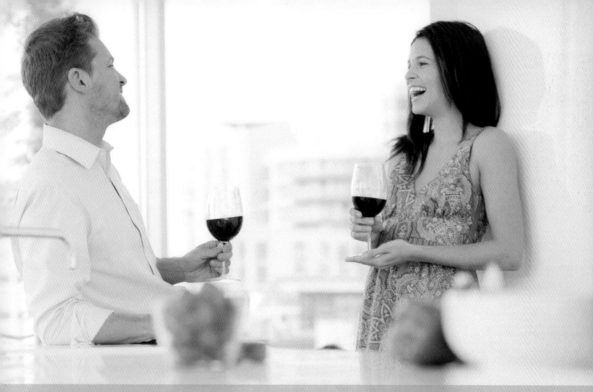

Red wine contains high concentrations of powerful antioxidants
– so a small glass a day does you good!

ANTIOXIDANT POWER

Red wine antioxidants inhibit the oxidation of 'bad' LDL-cholesterol and have a blood-thinning action to protect against hardening and furring-up of the arteries (atherosclerosis). The blood-thinning action is partly due to reduced levels of the blood-clotting factor fibrinogen, and partly due to an interaction with small circulating cell fragments, called platelets, which are also involved in the clotting process. Some dietary components, such as saturated fats, make platelets more sticky and promote platelet aggregation and clot formation, while others, such as marine fish oils, olive oil and red wine, inhibit platelet reactivity.

Plus, when red wine is consumed with meals, it is absorbed more slowly, prolonging this protective effect at a time when blood platelets are under the influence of dietary saturated fats. This is believed to be one of the underlying reasons for the French Paradox, and why wine drinkers in Sardinia, Crete and rural southwest France are among the healthiest, longest-lived people in the world.

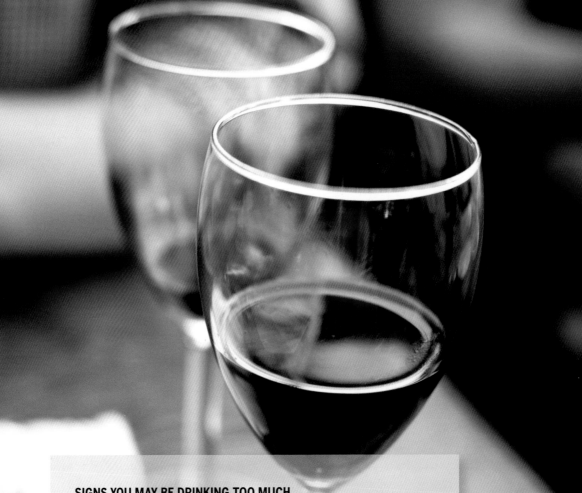

SIGNS YOU MAY BE DRINKING TOO MUCH

If you answer **YES** to any of the following questions, you may have
a problem with alcohol, and should speak to your doctor.

- Do you drink every day of the week?
- Do you ever feel you should cut down on your drinking?
- Do you ever need a drink first thing in the morning?
- Do you feel annoyed if people mention your drinking?
- Do you experience mood swings or difficulty sleeping after drinking?
- Do you feel hung over or shaky the morning after drinking?
- Do you ever miss work because of the effects of drinking?
- Do you drink and drive?

Artery disease Atherosclerosis is linked with the laying down of calcium in artery walls. Compared with non-drinkers, people who consume one drink per day have a 40 per cent reduction in extensive calcification of coronary arteries. Those who drink one to two alcoholic drinks per day have a 50 per cent reduction, but at higher intakes this protection is lost.

Moderation is key

Of course, the benefits of alcohol must be weighed against the harmful effects of excess. Heavy drinkers have an increased risk of high blood pressure and premature death from road traffic accidents, suicide, homicide, certain cancers (such as mouth, throat and breast), stroke, weakened heart muscle (cardiomyopathy) and cirrhosis of the liver.

WATCH YOUR CONSUMPTION

Men who regularly drink six units of alcohol per day (for example, six small glasses of wine or three pints of normal-strength beer) or who binge drink at weekends have almost twice the risk of sudden death due to heart-rhythm abnormalities than moderate or non-drinkers. In addition, excess alcohol lowers testosterone levels and hastens its conversion to oestrogen in the liver. Excessive intakes therefore lead to lowered sperm count and decreased sex drive, as well as erectile

DID YOU KNOW?

Moderate drinkers have a lower risk of dying if they do experience a heart attack, and a lower risk of experiencing a second heart attack in the future, than those who drink no alcohol.

problems. As much as 40 per cent of male infertility has been blamed on just a moderate intake of alcohol. Stopping drinking can improve sperm count within three months.

The adverse effects of excess alcohol are seen at lower doses in women, partly due to the increased risk of breast cancer associated with alcohol intake. Drinking more than two units of alcohol also lowers female oestrogen levels, and may lead to menstrual problems and lowered fertility. Women who drink five or less units of alcohol a week are twice as likely to conceive within six months, compared with women who regularly drink ten units per week or more.

Recent research suggests that the benefits of moderate alcohol intake do not apply equally to all people. Moderate drinking (one to two units per day) appears to be of most benefit for men over forty years of age and post-menopausal women.

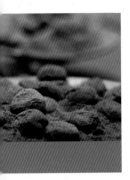

8 EAT dark chocolate

For many of us, chocolate is one of life's true pleasures, so it's a bonus to know that it offers unrivalled anti-ageing benefits, too – as long as it consists of at least 70 per cent cocoa solids.

Dark chocolate contains large quantities of antioxidant flavonoids – the same type that give red wine and green tea their heart-protecting reputation (*see* pages 46 and 58). What's more, the polyphenols present in chocolate are of the super-protective variety known as procyanidin flavonoids. While some of these flavonoids contain just one unit, and are classed as monomers, the most protective contain two, three or more units and are known as oligomers – and chocolate is especially rich in the larger oligomers that provide the greatest health benefits. In fact, the antioxidant potential of dark chocolate is higher than for just about any other superfood, at an extraordinary 103,971 ORAC units per 100 g. (For more on ORAC and the damaging effects of oxidation *see* pages 14 and 16.)

Championing chocolate

Chocolate antioxidants have beneficial effects throughout the body, especially the brain. It contains psychoactive compounds that include:

- **small amounts of caffeine** – around ten times less than the average cup of coffee, a concentration that is ideal for increasing alertness and decreasing perception of effort and fatigue, but without interfering with sleep
- **theobromine**, a caffeine-like stimulant which also peps you up
- **tryptophan**, an amino acid that acts as a building block for making serotonin, a brain chemical that lifts mood, increases euphoria and gives feelings of pleasure
- **a series of neuroactive alkaloids** that have an anti-cancer action by inhibiting an enzyme involved in uncontrolled cell division
- **phenylethylamine** (PEA) – a mood-altering substance (neuroamine) that has been described as the molecular basis for love; PEA is responsible for the initial feelings of swooning, walking on air and loss of appetite that accompany falling in love. PEA produces a mild, confidence-instilling buzz that intensifies feelings of pleasure; most chocolate-derived phenylethylamine is metabolized before it reaches the brain, but some people are sensitive to its effects in very small quantities

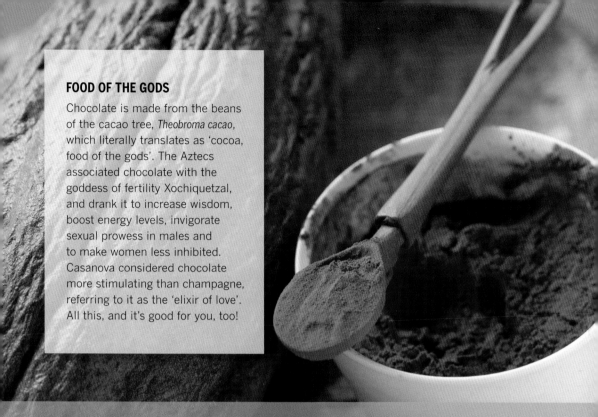

FOOD OF THE GODS

Chocolate is made from the beans of the cacao tree, *Theobroma cacao*, which literally translates as 'cocoa, food of the gods'. The Aztecs associated chocolate with the goddess of fertility Xochiquetzal, and drank it to increase wisdom, boost energy levels, invigorate sexual prowess in males and to make women less inhibited. Casanova considered chocolate more stimulating than champagne, referring to it as the 'elixir of love'. All this, and it's good for you, too!

Chocolate is especially rich in the type of flavonoids that provide the greatest health benefits for both body and mind.

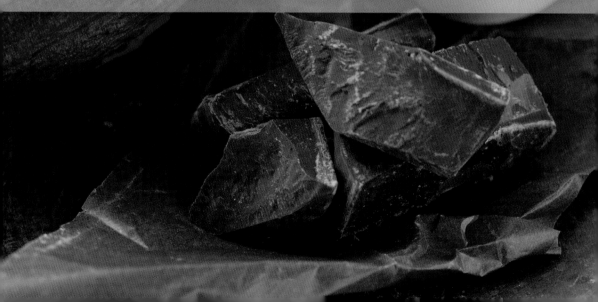

- **tiny amounts of anandamide**, an endogenous cannabinoid which stimulates the same brain receptors as marijuana; this contributes to feelings of contentment and contributes to a chocolate 'high'. Although you would need to eat several pounds of chocolate to obtain noticeable psychoactive effects, it's worth noting that chocolate also contains chemicals that inhibit the natural breakdown of anandamide, which means that eating chocolate makes you feel good for longer

Another plus point is that, like other agreeable sweet foods, consumption of chocolate also triggers the release of the body's own opiate-like endorphins that reduce sensitivity to pain.

Sexual function Researchers have suggested that chocolate may have a positive impact – either psychologically or biologically – on female sexuality. When urologists from San Raffaele hospital in Milan, Italy, questioned 163 women about their consumption of chocolate as well as their experience of sexual fulfilment, they found that the women who ate chocolate every day had significantly higher levels of desire than those who did not consume chocolate on a daily basis.

Heart disease Eating dark chocolate has been shown to improve a number of coronary-heart-disease risk factors. Research published in the *American Journal of Hypertension* showed that the high flavonoid content within 100 g (3½ oz) of dark chocolate has a beneficial effect on blood-vessel linings, reducing arterial stiffness, improving dilation and lowering blood pressure. Other scientists writing in the *British Medical Journal* agreed that eating 100 g of dark chocolate per day could reduce blood pressure by an average of 5.1/1.8 mmHg – enough to reduce the risk of a heart attack or stroke by 21 per cent. Interestingly, the Kuna Indians living on islands off the coast of Panama do not develop high blood pressure as they age, and this is partly attributed to the vast amounts of cocoa they consume daily.

Another heart-health benefit comes from cocoa butter, which is rich in monounsaturated oleic acid (the same type of fat that is found in olive oil). Dark chocolate has been shown to raise 'good' HDL-cholesterol levels while lowering 'bad' LDL-cholesterol by up to 10 per cent. Although cocoa butter also contains saturated fat, this is mostly in the form of stearic acid, which has a neutral effect on cholesterol levels.

DID YOU KNOW?

Women are more susceptible than men to the effects of chemicals such as PEA and tryptophan, and are therefore more likely to be chocoholics.

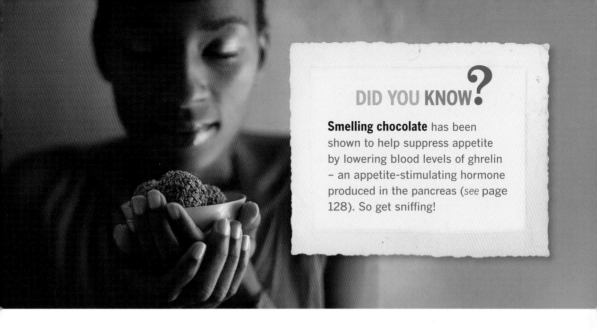

DID YOU KNOW?

Smelling chocolate has been shown to help suppress appetite by lowering blood levels of ghrelin – an appetite-stimulating hormone produced in the pancreas (see page 128). So get sniffing!

Dark chocolate also reduces unwanted platelet clumping and protects against blood clots – even in smokers. Researchers have also discovered that eating 45 g (1½ oz) dark chocolate a day significantly increases blood flow through the coronary arteries.

Diabetes Chocolate has also been shown to improve insulin sensitivity and pancreatic function in people with poor glucose tolerance, and this effect might even help to reduce the risk of developing type 2 diabetes.

LIVE LONGER

As a result of all these health benefits, researchers writing in the *British Journal of Medicine* predicted that including 100 g dark chocolate in your daily diet (along with regular intakes of fish, fruit, vegetables, almonds, garlic and 150 ml/5 fl oz wine) could potentially increase average life expectancy by six and a half years for men and five years for women. Drinking cocoa provides similar health benefits.

The downside

Unfortunately, chocolate does contain a lot of calories. The 100 g (3½ oz) of antioxidant-rich dark chocolate used in trials provides 510 kcal of energy which, if not worked off through increased exercise, could contribute to weight gain.

To get the most out of your anti-ageing chocolate 'medicine', make sure it's dark and contains at least 70 per cent cocoa solids – in fact, the darker, the better. Some brands now offer 90 and even 100 per cent cocoa solids – but the latter is so bitter it can usually only be eaten a single square at a time. Eat a little a day (up to a maximum of 100 g) as part of a balanced diet, in order to obtain some of the benefits without the additional fat and sugar.

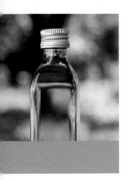

9 SWITCH TO olive oil

A key component of the Mediterranean diet (associated with one of the highest adult life expectancies in the world), olive oil can lower blood pressure, improve cholesterol balance and dramatically reduce the risk of a heart attack.

Populations following a Mediterranean diet tend to live longer than those following other patterns of eating. A number of studies have found that individuals who report eating foods consistent with the Mediterranean diet are 10 to 20 per cent less likely to die over the course of the study from heart disease, cancer or any other medical cause than those not consuming olive oil and other components of the diet.

DELICIOUS AND NUTRITIOUS

Hailing from Greece, Crete and Southern Italy, the Mediterranean diet combines large amounts of olive oil, vegetables, fruit, fish, garlic, wholegrains, beans, nuts, seeds, bread and potatoes, with a relatively low intake of red meat and a moderate consumption of red wine. Overall, the diet provides a total fat content of 25–35 per cent, with an unusually low intake of saturated fat that accounts for 8 per cent or less of energy intake.

Cooking with olive oil

According to researchers at the University of Münster, Germany, pure olive oil remains stable at elevated temperatures due to its high levels of monounsaturated fatty acids and the natural antioxidant, vitamin E. Refined olive oil can therefore be heated up to 210 C (410 F) before chemical changes take place. Virgin and extra virgin olive oils are less stable, however, due to the higher content of heat-sensitive components that contribute to their colour and flavour.

Because of this, virgin olive oil may cause unwanted smells or taste changes if heated above 180 C (350 F). So, only fry or roast with pure olive oil, and keep virgin or extra virgin olive oils for steaming, gentle braising and using in salad dressings.

As with other oils, oxidation occurs over time. Discard any oil that begins to smoke or smell odd during use. Cooking oils should not be re-used, as heat-altered oils are a source of toxic lipid peroxides, which are harmful to health.

Types of olive oil

Olive oil is derived from the fruit of the olive tree (*Olea europaea*), which is not considered fully productive until fifty to seventy-five years old. All olives start off green, as unripened fruit with a firm skin and slightly bitter taste. As the olive ripens, it passes through various shades of purple to black, and the flesh becomes increasingly wrinkled. The flavour also mellows as the oil content increases. Olives intended for producing oil are picked when unripe, as these have the lowest acid content and produce better oil.

Extra virgin olive oil is the best quality, as it has not been purified. Only around 10 per cent of oil produced is of this premium-grade quality. It has a distinctive green hue and often hazes at room temperature. Its flavour is superb, as it comes from the first pressing of the fruit and retains the fresh, olive aroma with less than one per cent acidity. It also has the highest antioxidant content (vitamin E, carotenoids and polyphenols).

Virgin olive oil comes next in quality, with an acidity level of not more than 1.5 per cent. Virgin olive oil is also a premium product, as it is not purified and is slightly more piquant in taste.

Pure olive oil (rather misleadingly) is a blend of refined oils mixed with virgin oil to provide flavour and a quality suitable for cooking. Acidity must be no more than 1.5 per cent and, although the flavour is less pleasing, this is the most widely sold oil, as it is less expensive. Many are processed with olive leaves to give a green colour that falsely mimics that of first-pressing, extra virgin olive oils.

STORING YOUR OIL

The major problem with olive oil is its rapid ageing. Most oils are best used within one year of pressing. If left longer, stale or even rancid flavours can develop – so don't lay down olive oil alongside your clarets! All types of olive oil should ideally be kept somewhere cool and dark, and used fresh – buy from outlets where turnover is high, and avoid large containers (especially those made from tin or aluminium). Olive oil can also be refrigerated for longer-term storage; it solidifies when chilled, but regains its liquidity and colour when returned to room temperature.

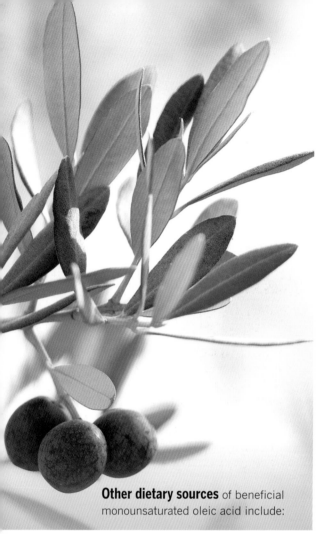

The healthy choice

Researchers have recently discovered that following a Mediterranean-style diet influences the activity of genes involved in the development and progression of hardening and furring-up of the arteries (atherosclerosis) and glucose control. Other benefits include:

Blood pressure Numerous studies show that a high olive oil intake reduces blood pressure. This is partly due to its antioxidants and partly due to its high oleic acid (OA) content, which is believed to be incorporated into cell membranes to trigger blood-vessel dilation. Among people with high blood pressure, using 30–40 g (1–1½ oz) olive oil for cooking every day halved the need for anti-hypertensive drugs over a six-month period, and 80 per cent were able to discontinue their drug treatment altogether (while those on a sunflower oil diet continued to need drug treatment). The blood-pressure-lowering effect is sufficient to reduce the risk of a stroke by up to 70 per cent.

Other dietary sources of beneficial monounsaturated oleic acid include:

TYPE OF OIL	% MONOUNSATURATED FAT
HAZELNUT	82
MACADAMIA NUT	81
OLIVE	73
ALMOND	68
AVOCADO	62
RAPESEED	60
PEANUT	44

Glucose control The monounsaturated fats, such as oleic acid, contained in olive oil have beneficial effects on insulin sensitivity. When people with type 2 diabetes replace some dietary carbohydrate with 10–40 g (¼–1½ oz) olive oil per day, their glucose control significantly improves, and it has been estimated that following an olive-oil-rich diet could potentially prevent over 90 per cent of cases of type 2 diabetes.

In a study involving 215 overweight people with newly diagnosed type 2 diabetes, one group followed an olive-oil-rich Mediterranean-style diet, while others followed a low-fat, low-calorie diet, or a relatively low-carbohydrate one. After four years, only 44 per cent of those on the Mediterranean-style diet needed to start taking glucose-lowering drugs, compared with 70 per cent in the other groups. They also lost more weight and showed greater improvements in other heart disease risk factors.

Cholesterol balance Consuming olive oil has beneficial effects on cholesterol balance, as it contains plant sterols that help block the absorption of cholesterol in the gut. It is also processed in the liver to lower the harmful LDL-cholesterol and raise 'good' HDL-cholesterol. These effects are greatest with virgin and extra virgin olive oils. A high-monounsaturated-fat diet also reduces blood levels of triglycerides (another type of fat).

Heart disease As a result of all these findings, doctors have estimated that combining regular exercise and not smoking with daily consumption of olive oil as part of a Mediterranean-style diet could prevent eight out of ten heart attacks and seven out of ten strokes. In the Lyon Diet Heart Study, for example, people who were asked to follow a Mediterranean-style diet after experiencing a heart attack were significantly less likely to have a second heart attack than those following a

MAKE IT MEDITERRANEAN
- Eat more fruit
- Eat more vegetables, beans and potatoes
- Eat more nuts and seeds
- Use olive oil rather than other cooking/ dressing oils
- Select wholegrain bread and cereals
- Eat more fish
- Eat low to moderate amounts of dairy produce and poultry
- Eat only a little red meat
- Eat no more than four eggs a week
- Consume wine in low to moderate amounts

'prudent Western-type diet'. In fact, the protective effects were so striking – a 70 per cent reduction in death – that the study was stopped after twenty-seven months (rather than the planned five years), as it was thought unethical not to advise those in the control group to also follow a Mediterranean way of eating.

Cellular ageing One of the main causes of ageing is damage to our genetic material (DNA). This is especially true within structures called mitochondria, which act as the cell's batteries. Researchers suggest that consuming more monounsaturated fats such as olive oil and cutting back on total polyunsaturated fats (especially omega-6s) can protect our DNA. Monounsaturated fats are less prone to oxidation, and so trigger less of the inflammatory reactions that damage DNA and result in age-related mutations.

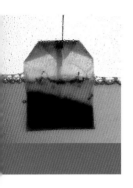

10 DRINK MORE tea

Tea is one of the most popular drinks in the world – and it's good for us, too! Drinking just four cups a day can halve your risk of a heart attack, and tea drinkers are also less likely to suffer from high blood pressure and stroke.

The origins of tea-drinking are lost in the mists of time. An ancient Chinese legend claims that tea was introduced as a beverage in 2737 BCE, but the earliest confirmed reference to the cultivation, processing and drinking of tea is to be found in a Chinese dictionary dating from the fourth century CE.

The health benefits of tea have long been well known in China, where it was considered a medicinal beverage and often referred to as 'Tai fu', which means 'doctor'.

DID YOU KNOW?

White tea contains around 15 mg caffeine per cup, compared to 20 mg for green tea and 40 mg for black tea – so if you're trying to cut down on your caffeine consumption, go for white or green.

What's in your cuppa?

Tea is composed of the young leaves and leaf buds of the shrub *Camellia sinensis*. Two main varieties are used: the small-leaved China tea plant (*C. sinensis sinensis*) and the large-leaved Assam tea plant (*C. sinensis assamica*).

Green tea is made by steaming and drying fresh tea leaves immediately after harvesting, while the more familiar black tea is made by crushing and fermenting freshly cut tea leaves so that they oxidize before drying. This allows natural enzymes in the tea leaves to produce the characteristic red-brown colour and also serves to reduce astringency.

White tea is similar to green tea, in that it's not fermented, but it is only made from new tea buds, picked before they open. These have a white appearance due to the presence of fine, silvery hairs. The buds are gently dried and make a tea that is pale, straw-coloured and delicately fragrant – described as light and sweet. White tea doesn't develop the characteristic 'grassy' flavour of green tea (which can be an acquired taste), yet it's just

The humble cup of tea can reduce the risk of a heart attack or stroke, as well as boost our resistance to infection.

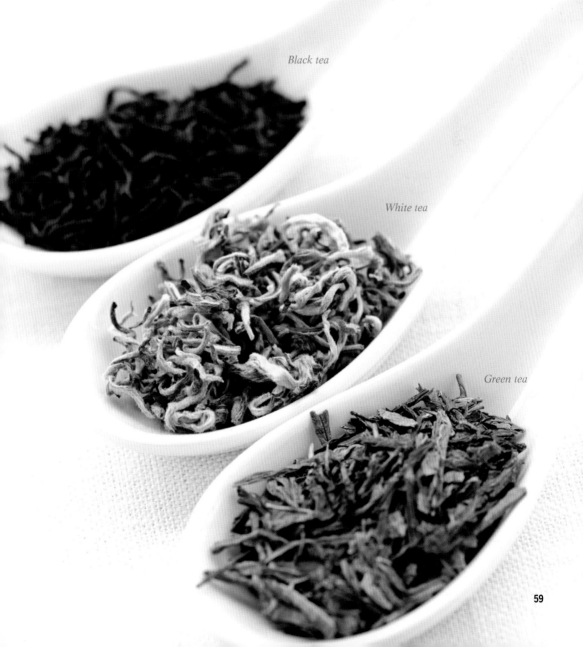

Black tea

White tea

Green tea

> Drinking four to five cups of black tea per day provides more than half of our total dietary intake of flavonoid antioxidants.

as beneficial for our health, which may be why it's now becoming increasingly popular in the West. Black tea currently accounts for around 75 per cent of the world's tea consumption, mainly in the West, while green tea – the most popular tea in Asian countries – accounts for the majority of the remainder.

FANTASTIC FLAVONOIDS

Over 30 per cent of the dry weight of green tea leaves consists of powerful flavonoid antioxidants such as catechins. These are converted into less active antioxidants (such as theaflavins and thearubigins) during fermentation, but even so, drinking four to five cups of black tea per day provides over 50 per cent of our total dietary intake of flavonoid antioxidants (with the other 50 per cent coming mainly from apples and onions).

Antioxidants such as those found in tea are also known to help maintain healthy circulation, bones and teeth, as well as boosting our resistance to infection. They are also important in the fight against premature ageing – so much so that green tea extracts are now being added to some cosmetics to help maintain youthful skin, hair and nails.

Put the kettle on

When you make yourself a cup of tea, it's more than just a refreshing brew that you're enjoying …

Coronary heart disease Research suggests that drinking green tea has beneficial effects on blood cholesterol balance, blood pressure and blood stickiness, and can decrease the risk of coronary heart disease. People who drink at least four cups of tea a day are half as likely to experience a heart attack as non-tea drinkers, and are also less likely to suffer from high blood pressure and stroke. A recent large analysis of data from eighteen studies showed that drinking just one cup of green tea per day can lower the risk of coronary heart disease by 10 per cent. Previous studies suggest that drinking black tea is also beneficial, with three or more cups of tea improving antioxidant status and providing some protection against heart disease.

Cancer High intakes (around eight to ten cups a day) of green tea are thought to protect against cancers of the liver, ovary, womb and lung, and possibly the stomach and colon, too. In addition, analysis of results from four studies

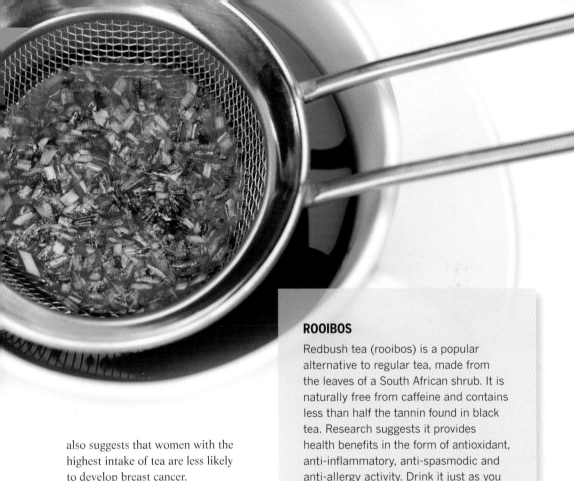

also suggests that women with the highest intake of tea are less likely to develop breast cancer.

Weight loss Extracts from green tea leaves can boost the rate at which the body burns calories by as much as 40 per cent over a 24-hour period. This is due to its ability to inhibit a particular metabolic enzyme, so that levels of noradrenaline increase to stimulate the amount of energy burned in body cells (thermogenesis). It may also block the activity of intestinal enzymes needed to digest dietary fat, so that less fat is absorbed. Several trials have suggested that adding green tea extracts to a

ROOIBOS

Redbush tea (rooibos) is a popular alternative to regular tea, made from the leaves of a South African shrub. It is naturally free from caffeine and contains less than half the tannin found in black tea. Research suggests it provides health benefits in the form of antioxidant, anti-inflammatory, anti-spasmodic and anti-allergy activity. Drink it just as you would black tea, with or without milk, sugar or lemon.

weight loss regime helps to improve fat loss. For example, a study involving sixty obese adults following a prepared diet of three meals a day found that, compared with placebo, those taking green tea extracts lost an additional 2.7 kg (6 lb) during the first month, 5.1 kg (11¼ lb) during the second month and 3.3 kg (7¼ lb) during the third month.

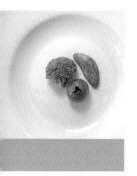

11 EAT less overall

Studies suggest that restricting calorie intake can extend our lifespan, as well as reducing blood pressure, lowering cholesterol and even benefiting neurological conditions such as Alzheimer's and Parkinson's.

Most of us eat too much to achieve longevity. Studies carried out on a variety of animal species, including fish, mice, rats, dogs and monkeys, suggest that prolonged restriction of calorie intake can significantly extend lifespan by 50–100 per cent. And, while long-term studies on calorie restriction in humans are still in progress, it is believed that, in all likelihood, following a restricted diet can extend human life, too.

A recent review published in *Psychology & Behaviour* even stated that calorie restriction (while maintaining proper nutrition) is the only intervention known to consistently decrease the biological rate of ageing and to increase both average and maximal lifespan. Unfortunately, you need to restrict calorie intake to around two-thirds of your normal daily needs in order to prolong your life by twenty to forty years and, for those gourmands who enjoy their food, this might well be too high a price to pay.

DID YOU KNOW?

In Japan, longevity is sought through a philosophy of dietary restriction known as *hara hachi bu* or 'eight parts out of ten', in which followers eat only until they are 80 per cent full – an ideal way to prevent over-eating!

Longevity in practice

The best evidence for calorie restriction prolonging human life currently comes from those living on the Japanese island of Okinawa, where there are five times more centenarians in the population (fifty per 100,000 people) compared with most industrialized countries. Their exceptional longevity has been attributed to their traditional, vegetable-rich diet, which is low in calories but high in vitamins, minerals and antioxidants (*see* page 22). This low-calorie intake was first observed in schoolchildren on Okinawa more than forty years ago, and later studies confirm that, on average, Okinawan adults eat 20 per cent fewer calories than those living on mainland Japan.

ALTERNATE EATING

Eating every other day (fasting one day, and eating what you like the next) appears to produce similar effects, with health benefits becoming apparent within as little as two weeks. Researchers writing in the journal *Medical Hypotheses* suggested this strategy might improve insulin resistance, asthma, allergies, infections, autoimmune diseases, osteoarthritis, heart problems and menopausal symptoms. It may also delay, prevent or improve neurological conditions such as Alzheimer's, Parkinson's and multiple sclerosis.

In one early study involving 120 men, half were allowed to eat whatever they wanted, while the other group fasted on alternate days for three years. Over this period they ate, on average, 1500 kcal per day – a 35 per cent calorie restriction compared with the control group. Over the next twenty years, those subjected to calorie restriction were half as likely to be admitted to hospital or to die than those who ate every day.

So how does it work?

Calorie restriction has been associated with lower cholesterol and triglyceride levels, reduced blood pressure and improved glucose control, as well as prevention or delay in the development of neurological conditions such as those mentioned above. And, while it is not yet fully understood why severe calorie restriction without malnutrition extends lifespan, for these reasons prolonged life is thought to result from a number of significant changes in energy metabolism, oxidative damage, insulin sensitivity, inflammation, hormone secretion and nervous-system activity.

WHAT THE FACTS SHOW

A study called CALERIE (Comprehensive Assessment of the Long-term Effect of Reducing Intake of Energy) is currently ongoing in the US to test the effects of a 25 per cent calorie restriction in non-obese healthy men and women aged between twenty-five and forty-five. In the first phase of the trial, one group is eating only 75 per cent of their

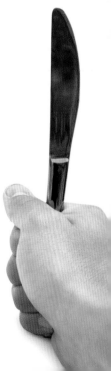

Restricting calorie intake has been shown to decrease biological rate of ageing and prolong lifespan.

estimated calorie requirement (in other words, a 25 per cent calorie restriction), while another group is also achieving a 25 per cent calorie restriction but half of this is being met by increasing their level of exercise. A third group is following a low-calorie diet of 890 kcal per day to achieve a 15 per cent weight loss, and will then follow a weight maintenance diet, while a fourth control group is following a healthy diet designed to maintain their current weight.

After six months, both groups following the 25 per cent calorie restriction showed a 10 per cent fall in body weight, with significant reductions in fat mass (24 per cent), visceral fat (27 per cent) and a reduction in liver fat (27 per cent), suggesting that exercise and calorie restriction play equivalent roles in terms of energy balance. Their blood pressure reduced and 'good' HDL-cholesterol increased enough to reduce their risk of experiencing a heart attack over the next ten years by 28 per cent. Body temperature and thyroid hormone levels also reduced, so that their metabolic rate decreased 6 per cent more than expected from their loss of

body mass alone. As a result, they generated significantly fewer oxidation reactions (which bombard cells and genetic material). As oxidation reactions are one of the leading causes of premature ageing, this is potentially one of the greatest anti-ageing effects of calorie restriction (*see* Combating Oxidation, page 14).

Less is more

If cutting out around a quarter of your daily calorie intake sounds like a step too far – which is probably the case for most of us! – there are still easy things you can do to adjust your eating habits (especially if you have a tendency to over-indulge). Eating even just a little less each day can do wonders for long-term health and well-being, and you'll feel all the better for it.

Try these tips (and *see also* page 70):
- It takes about 20 minutes for your brain to register that you're full – so aim to stop when you reach the Okinawans' magic 80 per cent, and you should feel sated soon after.
- Try eating at a more leisurely pace, so that your brain has a chance to catch up with your stomach.
- Don't over-fill your plate (it can be difficult to stop eating when you've only got a few mouthfuls left, even if you're already fit to burst).
- If you're tempted to go back for seconds, give it a few minutes and the urge will most likely pass.

CAUTION!

If restricting calories, take a multivitamin and mineral supplement to ensure adequate intake of vitamins and minerals.

Very-low-calorie diets

A number of very-low-calorie diets (VLCDs) are available for weight loss. These typically provide between 400 and 800 kcal per day in the form of fortified, sweet or savoury drinks that replace between one and three meals daily. These provide the vitamins and minerals you need but significantly restrict your energy intake. Under professional supervision, these diets can help you lose between 13 and 23 kg (29 to 51 lb) excess weight.

Although these diets used to be considered extreme, they are now gaining medical acceptance for some people as part of an ongoing, structured education and behavioural-support programme to change long-term eating and lifestyle habits. A large analysis of twenty-nine studies, investigating how well people managed to keep excess weight off once they had lost it, found that VLCDs were markedly more successful than a traditional calorie-controlled or low-fat diet, and helped people keep off significantly more weight at every year of follow-up – even up to five years later.

MEDICAL ADVICE

Potentially, these VLCDs could be adapted to help people of a healthy weight restrict their calorie intake, if they choose, in order to live longer. However, there is a caveat. People with a body mass index (BMI – *see* page 67) of less than 18.5 are considered underweight, which brings its own health problems associated with reduced immunity, hormone imbalances, nutritional deficiencies and eating disorders. If you decide to follow a calorie-restricted diet, it is therefore important to do so only under the advice of a qualified dietician or nutritionist – and preferably one who has extensive medical training and experience.

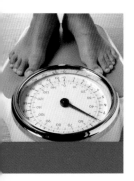

12 MAINTAIN A
healthy weight

Keeping your weight within the healthy weight range for your height helps to reduce the risk of heart disease, stroke, high blood pressure, diabetes and even some types of cancer.

It's common – even normal – for us to gain weight as we age. This mostly comes from age-related reductions in lean muscle mass, and a slowing of your metabolic rate. Most people don't reduce their calorie intake or increase their level of physical activity to compensate for this – in fact, more often than not, retirement means that food intake increases and exercise levels reduce.

Unfortunately, carrying excess weight is associated with significant health risks. Obesity:
- increases the risk of type 2 diabetes almost forty-fold, especially when excess fat is deposited around your abdomen
- doubles the risk of dying prematurely from coronary heart disease and stroke
- doubles your risk of developing asthma

As a result, someone who is obese will die, on average, seven years earlier than someone in the healthy weight range for their height, while those who are severely obese are twelve times more likely to die prematurely.

Why excess fat is harmful

Being overweight tends to be associated with unhealthy lifestyles such as a high-fat diet and lack of exercise – but our genes are also involved. Our ancestors evolved on a frugal diet with frequent periods of famine. Those able to conserve energy and store fat survived best, and these genes – selected by evolutionary pressures to help our ancestors survive – are now counting against us.

People who inherit genes that deposit excess fat around the internal organs (referred to as 'apple-shaped')

Losing excess weight reduces your risk of developing common age-related problems, helping you stay healthier for longer.

Calculating your Body Mass Index (BMI)

Your body-fat stores can be estimated using a calculation in which you divide your weight (in kilograms) by your height in metres squared. (If you're converting from imperial measurements, 2.2 lb is equivalent to 1 kg. Check the table below to find your height in metres.)

$$BMI = \frac{weight\ (kg)}{height\ (m) \times height\ (m)}$$

This produces a number called your Body Mass Index (BMI), which indicates your weight classification (see below).

HEIGHT		OPTIMUM HEALTHY WEIGHT RANGE	
metres	feet	kilograms	pounds
1.47	4'10"	40.0 – 53.8	88 – 119
1.50	4'11"	41.6 – 56.0	92 – 123
1.52	5'0"	42.7 – 57.5	94 – 127
1.55	5'1"	44.4 – 59.8	98 – 132
1.57	5'2"	45.6 – 61.4	100 – 135
1.60	5'3"	47.4 – 63.7	104 – 140
1.63	5'4"	49.2 – 66.2	108 – 145
1.65	5'5"	50.4 – 66.6	111 – 147
1.68	5'6"	52.2 – 70.3	115 – 155
1.70	5'7"	53.5 – 72.0	118 – 159
1.73	5'8"	55.4 – 74.5	122 – 164
1.75	5'9"	56.7 – 76.3	125 – 168
1.78	5'10"	58.6 – 78.9	129 – 174
1.80	5'11"	60.0 – 80.7	132 – 178
1.83	6'0"	62.0 – 83.4	137 – 184
1.85	6'1"	63.3 – 85.2	140 – 188
1.88	6'2"	65.4 – 88.0	144 – 194
1.90	6'3"	66.8 – 89.9	147 – 198
1.93	6'4"	68.9 – 92.8	152 – 205

CLASSIFICATION	BMI (kg/m²)
Underweight	under 18.5
Normal range	18.5 to 24.9
Overweight (pre-obese)	25 to 29.9
Obese	30 to 39.9
Severely obese	40 or greater

The table above shows the healthy weight range for adults, according to height. If you're within the range for your height, then you do not have an excess risk of dying prematurely as a result of your weight.

are more likely to develop health problems than those who store fat around their hips ('pear-shaped'). This is because visceral (intra-abdominal) fat is different from fat stored elsewhere in the body. It secretes hormones and free fatty acids that travel directly to your liver. Here, they activate genes that increase liver production of cholesterol, clotting factors and other inflammatory chemicals that make blood more sticky and raise your blood pressure. These chemicals also act as a signal that fat stores are full, so cells become resistant to the effects of insulin and less glucose can enter cells. In addition, when free-fatty-acid levels are high, muscle cells burn them – rather than glucose – as a fuel.

All these factors contribute to impaired glucose tolerance and significantly increase your risk of type 2 diabetes. The inflammation associated with obesity also increases the risk of heart attack, stroke and several cancers, including those of the breast, uterus and colon.

Losing excess weight

Your daily energy requirement depends on your age, gender, level of activity and occupation. The average daily energy needs for men and women are shown in the table below. To lose excess weight, you need to consume less energy than you require, so that the deficit is met by raiding your body-fat stores.

Losing 10 kg (22 lb) of excess fat can reduce your risk of premature death by 20 per cent and your risk of a diabetes-related death by as much as 30 per cent. These benefits occur because a 10 kg fat loss improves several different risk factors:

- blood pressure falls by, on average, 10/20 mmHg
- fasting blood glucose levels improve by 50 per cent
- triglyceride levels (blood fats) fall by around 30 per cent
- total cholesterol levels decrease by 10 per cent
- harmful LDL-cholesterol falls by 15 per cent, while 'good' HDL-cholesterol increases by at least 8 per cent

AGE	MALES (kcal)	FEMALES (kcal)
15–18 years	2755	2110
19–50 years	2550	1940
51–59 years	2550	1900
60–64 years	2380	1900
65–74 years	2330	1900
75+ years	2100	1810

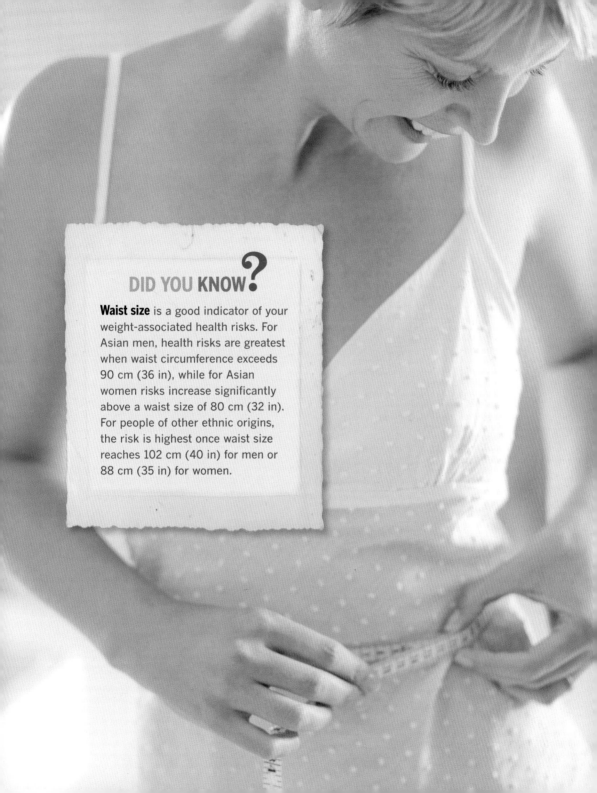

DID YOU KNOW?

Waist size is a good indicator of your weight-associated health risks. For Asian men, health risks are greatest when waist circumference exceeds 90 cm (36 in), while for Asian women risks increase significantly above a waist size of 80 cm (32 in). For people of other ethnic origins, the risk is highest once waist size reaches 102 cm (40 in) for men or 88 cm (35 in) for women.

Even slight waist reductions of just 5–10 cm (2–4 in) can significantly reduce your risk of a heart attack.

EXERCISE FOR SUCCESS

Sadly, losing weight is easier said than done. A number of hormones actively promote appetite and work against weight loss, including ghrelin (made in the pancreas – *see* page 128) and cortisol, produced in the adrenal glands during times of stress. Cortisol puts the body on 'red alert' and conserves energy by reducing the breakdown of body-fat stores. Unfortunately, going on a crash diet is exactly the kind of physical stress that triggers production of cortisol, which is one reason why dieting often doesn't work.

Exercise helps to overcome the effects of cortisol by resetting the fight-or-flight stress reaction to the rest-and-digest response. It also boosts fat-burning, reduces insulin resistance and triggers the release of endorphins – brain chemicals that suppress hunger and increase feelings of euphoria. Exercise is therefore an important part of any weight loss programme (*see* pages 72–5).

Dieting decisions

So what type of diet is best? Regrettably, there's no magic answer to this question. Opinions vary as to the most effective type of weight loss diet, and the success of a diet often differs from one person to another, too. A Gold-standard (Cochrane) review, for example, found that overweight and obese people following a low-glycemic diet (*see* page 128) lost more weight than those following other types of diet (low-fat, low-calorie), regardless of whether calorie intake was restricted or they were allowed to eat as much as they wished. Another trial, on the other hand, concluded that following a Mediterranean-style diet (*see* pages 56–7) or a low-glycemic diet may be more effective than a low-fat diet.

KEY RULES

Whichever type of diet you follow, it's important that any weight you lose is fat rather than lean muscle. It comes down to two main things: eat less and exercise more. Adopting the following habits should help, too:

- **Always eat breakfast** to kick-start your metabolism, so you burn more energy.
- **Drink a glass of water before eating** to help you fill up and avoid mistaking thirst for hunger.
- **Always sit down at a laid table;** eating while doing other things means you won't appreciate what you're eating and may eat more.
- **Use a smaller plate**, so you think you're eating more than you actually are.
- **Serve smaller helpings** than you think you need – more often than not, our eyes are bigger than our stomach.
- **Don't leave serving dishes on the table** or you're likely to serve too much – and go back for more, too!

- **Chew each mouthful for longer** to give your brain more time to receive signals that you're becoming full.
- **Pause regularly while eating**, so your meal lasts longer and you start to feel full up before you've eaten too much.
- **Purposely leave some food on your plate** – don't scrape your plate clean.
- **Wait to eat:** to tell hunger and appetite apart, force yourself to wait an extra 15–20 minutes whenever you fancy a snack. If it was appetite, the urge will disappear; if it was true hunger, sit down at the table and eat a healthy snack.
- **Keep a food diary** and write down everything you eat – this is especially helpful if you're finding it difficult to lose weight.

Eating breakfast kick-starts your metabolism, meaning that you burn more energy.

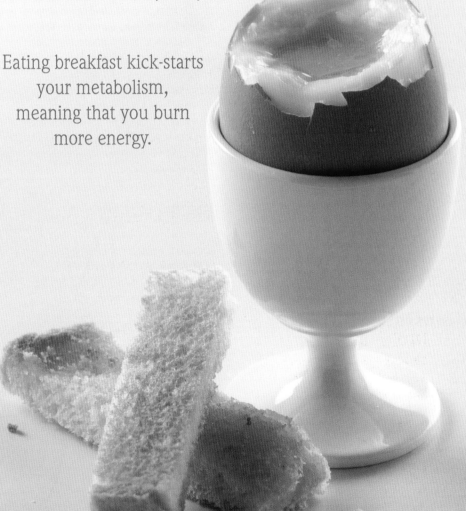

71

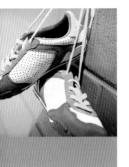

13 EXERCISE every day

Regular daily exercise has been shown to reduce the number of age-related deaths – from all medical causes – by almost a quarter, even if exercise is not started until middle age. So it's not too late to do something about it!

Regular exercise promotes good control of blood pressure, cholesterol balance, glucose levels and blood stickiness, and reduces the risk of developing most age-related diseases. In fact, taking regular exercise appears to offer as great a protection against premature death as not smoking.

A recent large study (published in *The Lancet*), which followed more than 416,000 men and women aged twenty and over for an eight-year period, showed that taking as little as 15 minutes of physical activity a day (or 90 minutes per week) reduced the risk of dying prematurely by 14 per cent and increased lifespan by three years.

Those who exercised more enjoyed greater benefits, with each additional 15 minutes of daily exercise further reducing their risk of death, from any medical cause, by another 4 per cent. This trend continued until the level of exercise reached 100 minutes, after which no further benefit was seen. Interestingly, vigorous activity for short periods of time had the same beneficial effect as less intense exercise carried out for longer.

Healthy activity

The health benefits of physical activity appear to result from immediate biological responses that persist for a short time after each exercise session, rather than from training effects. By exercising daily, these short-term benefits can be prolonged.

Cancer In the study quoted above, those who took just 15 minutes exercise per day were 11 per cent less likely to die from cancer during the course of the study than those who were inactive. And the risk of dying

DIABETES DEFENCE

The number of glucose receptors available to allow glucose to enter muscle cells is twice as high in those who train regularly, compared with those who lead a sedentary lifestyle.

from cancer continued to fall by 1 per cent for each additional 15 minutes of daily exercise on top of this.

Blood pressure Although exercise itself increases blood pressure, this falls as soon as you stop, through effects on blood-vessel dilation. This reduces blood pressure at rest and in situations that typically elevate blood pressure, such as further intense physical activity and emotional distress. Studies suggest that exercise reduces average blood pressures by 6–13 mmHg for the first 16 hours after exercise, compared to a day without exercise. Regular exercise, preferably on a daily basis, is therefore needed to maintain these benefits.

Blood fats Hardening and furring-up of the arteries is now recognized as linked with rises in blood-fat levels (triglycerides, LDL-cholesterol), blood stickiness and changes in blood flow that occur after eating. Regular exercise has beneficial effects against all these

variables, as it boosts liver function and increases the amount of fat broken down for use as a fuel. People who train every day have significantly lower peaks in blood-fat levels after eating compared with those who don't exercise daily, although their blood levels after fasting are similar. These beneficial effects are also short-lived, so exercising on most days is needed to maintain them. The good news, however, is that the 30

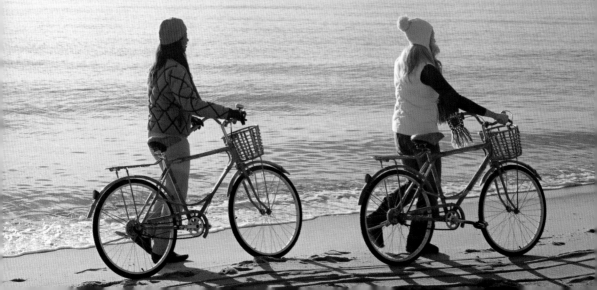

minutes' brisk walking per day is equally effective when accumulated throughout the day, rather than taken in one continuous session.

Weight Exercise boosts metabolic rate by as much as ten times, so you burn more calories even at rest. People who store fat round their internal organs and waist – the so-called 'apple' shape – are at increased risk of developing high blood pressure and diabetes. This type of fat, known as visceral fat, is readily reduced by exercise. Following a controlled jogging, rowing or cycling regime for 45 minutes, three days a week, has been shown to reduce weight by around 3 per cent over the course of a year – even if you don't change your eating habits – with most fat lost from around the waist and no increase in muscle mass.

Glucose control Exercise increases the amount of glucose taken up into muscle cells. Physical activity therefore plays an important role in preventing type 2 diabetes, with the greatest protective effect seen in those with highest risk. Both the Finnish Diabetes Prevention Study and the Diabetes Prevention Program showed that overweight subjects with impaired glucose tolerance could reduce their chance of progressing to type 2 diabetes by 58 per cent if they made lifestyle changes that included at least 150 minutes' physical activity per week (such as cycling, skiing, swimming, resistance training and snow-shovelling). For those of us who prefer something a little more low-key, low-intensity leisure activity, including gardening and walking, was also shown to be beneficial, and those who increased the intensity of their walking reduced their risk of progressing to type 2 diabetes by almost half, compared with those who did not.

A large analysis of data from fourteen trials has also shown that regular exercise improves glycemic control in those who have already developed type 2 diabetes. The beneficial effects of exercise on glucose tolerance only last for around three days, however, so regular exercise is needed to maintain these benefits.

Activate your daily routine

Exercise needs to occur on an almost daily basis to maintain acute, short-term benefits on blood pressure, blood-fat levels and glucose tolerance. But the good news is that physical activity doesn't have to be vigorous to benefit health: brisk walking for 30 to 60 minutes a day, most days a week, is associated with significant reductions in age-related health risks (even if you can only manage 15 minutes a day, that's better than nothing!).

There are plenty of other ways to increase your daily level of activity, too, without feeling as though you're working out. Gardening, doing housework or DIY, walking to the shops – it all makes a difference. Or, for exercise that doesn't feel like a chore, investigate taking up an active hobby like dancing, bowling or even a martial art. If you have a sedentary job, move around as much as you can during the day – go for a walk at lunchtime, or go and talk to a colleague in person, for instance, instead of phoning or emailing them from your desk. Do whatever you can to stay active.

Here are some useful habits to adopt, to make exercise part of your daily routine:
- Walk (or jog) upstairs, instead of taking the lift or escalator.
- Get off the bus or train one or two stops early and walk briskly the rest of the way.

STEP IT UP

Research shows that walking 10,000 steps a day can significantly improve our health, so clip a pedometer to your clothes to count the number of paces you take, and do your best to achieve this magic target.

- If you're driving somewhere, park the car a little way away from your destination, so that you still get a brief walk (or, better still, cycle instead!).

TAKING IT FURTHER

Once you are relatively fit, aim to do more. Exercise briskly enough to raise your pulse above 100 beats per minute, raise a light sweat and make you slightly breathless – but not so much that you can't hold a conversation. Adding resistance training (which uses weights) to aerobic exercise can enhance insulin sensitivity, decrease waist circumference and increase muscle density more than a similar quantity of aerobic training alone. This means either buying dumb-bells and other home exercise equipment, or joining a local gym for professional guidance.

If you are in any doubt about the level of exercise you can tolerate, seek advice from your doctor.

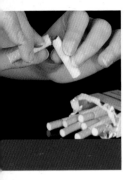

14 STOP smoking

Smoking is the single greatest cause of preventable death across the globe. Quitting almost immediately halves your risk of a heart attack or stroke and, in time, can reduce the risk of lung cancer and heart attack to normal levels.

More than one billion people smoke cigarettes worldwide, an estimated 5 million of whom die every year as a direct result of the habit. According to the World Health Organization, another 1,000 million will die a smoking-related death during this century. In fact, the reduction in mortality due to not smoking is so great that being a non-smoker can add an estimated fourteen years to your lifespan.

What smoking does

Cigarettes are harmful because the burning of tobacco leaves exposes you to over 4,000 different chemicals, of which at least sixty are carcinogenic and four hundred are toxic. These chemicals cause a great deal of damage to your:

- **airways**, increasing the risk of asthma, pneumonia, chronic bronchitis and emphysema
- **genetic material**, to trigger many cancers
- **artery linings**, to hasten hardening and furring-up of the arteries, high blood pressure, abnormal blood clotting and arterial spasm
- **pancreatic cell function**, to increase the chance of developing diabetes by as much as five times
- **kidney function**, to increase the risk of developing kidney failure
- **blood vessels in the eye**, to increase the risk of visual loss

DID YOU KNOW?

Every time you smoke a cigarette, your blood pressure can rise by 9/8 mmHg. This is thought to result from nicotine-induced stimulation of the sympathetic nervous system, which causes arterial constriction. If you smoke a cigarette and drink coffee at the same time, the increase is even greater – in some people, as high as 21/17 mmHg.

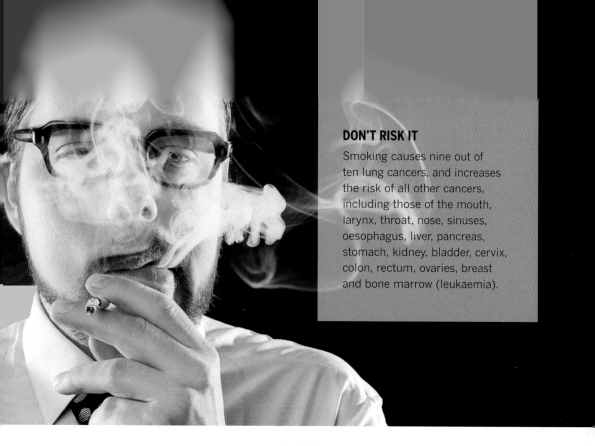

DON'T RISK IT

Smoking causes nine out of ten lung cancers, and increases the risk of all other cancers, including those of the mouth, larynx, throat, nose, sinuses, oesophagus, liver, pancreas, stomach, kidney, bladder, cervix, colon, rectum, ovaries, breast and bone marrow (leukaemia).

Overall, smoking increases your risk of a heart attack seven-fold and quadruples your risk of a stroke. By reducing blood flow to the peripheries, it is also associated with gangrene and limb amputation. In addition, one in two smokers dies of a smoking-related cancer.

Most smokers develop two or more smoking-related illnesses within their lifetime, and half of all smoking-related premature deaths occur during middle age. Low-tar brands aren't much safer, as they still contain other harmful chemicals such as benzene, ammonia, acetone, arsenic, cyanide and formaldehyde.

Quitting

The nicotine that is released from burning tobacco leaves is highly addictive. Withdrawal symptoms of tension, aggression, depression, insomnia and both physical and psychological cravings make it difficult to quit. If you successfully stop smoking, however, the stickiness of your blood will improve enough within 48 hours to halve your risk of a heart attack or stroke. Within five years, your risk of developing lung cancer will also halve and, within ten years, reduce to normal levels. After fifteen years, your risk of a heart attack will also have

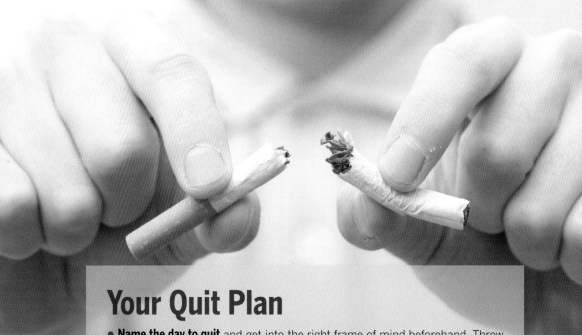

Your Quit Plan

- **Name the day to quit** and get into the right frame of mind beforehand. Throw away all smoking-related items such as cigarettes, rolling-papers, matches, lighters and ashtrays.

- **Find support**, as it's easier to quit together with a friend or relative who also wants to give up.

- **Take it one day at a time.** Think positively and concentrate on getting through Today. Keeping a Quit Chart and ticking off each cigarette-free day can help – don't focus on the weeks and months ahead.

- **Keep your hands busy** with a stress-relief ball, or try drawing, model-making, crochet, knitting or home repairs. These activities help to overcome the psychological hand-to-mouth habit that makes quitting so difficult.

- **Use artificial cigarettes, carrot or celery sticks** if the hand-to-mouth habit is difficult to overcome.

- **Exercise regularly** to increase your production of opium-like brain endorphins, to help curb withdrawal symptoms.

- **Reward yourself** at the end of the first day, week, month, and so on. Putting aside the money you save by not smoking can even pay for a holiday after as little as six months.

- **Avoid situations where you used to smoke.** Learn to say, 'No thanks, I've given up' or 'No thanks, I'm cutting down.'

reduced down to the same level as that of non-smokers. As a result, those who stop smoking in middle age have a good chance of avoiding a smoking-related premature death. And, quitting means you protect those around you from the harmful effects of passive smoking, too.

Most people are able to become a non-smoker within three months, and those who make a Quit Plan (*see* opposite) are twice as likely to succeed as those who just stop without thinking things through properly first.

NICOTINE REPLACEMENT THERAPY

The physical cravings caused by nicotine usually disappear within seven days, but the psychological 'need' lasts longer. Obtaining nicotine alone is significantly less harmful than inhaling it along with the 4,000 other chemicals present in tobacco smoke, so nicotine replacement therapy (NRT) is therefore an effective way to help manage cravings and withdraw from cigarette smoking. The quit rate with NRT is two to three times higher than for those who try to give up unaided. Electronic cigarettes provide nicotine in a familiar way and can help smokers quit.

CAUTION!

Nicotine receptors throughout the body can cause side effects, which include headache, dizziness, palpitations, nausea, abdominal pain, diarrhoea and weakness, among others. The minimum lethal dose of nicotine for a non-tolerant man is estimated at around 40 mg, so it's not a drug to use lightly; smoking while using an NRT product may lead to a harmful nicotine overdose.

Don't be tempted to use NRT while still smoking, and, if using nicotine replacement, monitor your blood pressure closely. If you are unsure about using NRT, ask your doctor for advice.

OTHER USEFUL METHODS

Other options may be helpful, too:

● **Hypnotherapy** can help one in three people quit smoking, though not everyone is susceptible to hypnotic suggestion.

● **Antidepressant drugs** such as bupropion or nortriptyline may be prescribed to help you quit smoking. Their effectiveness appears to be similar to that of NRT.

It's not too late: quitting in middle age can reduce your health risks back to normal levels.

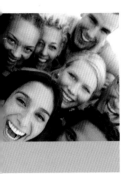

15 BE MORE sociable

Friends are good for you! According to psychologists, our relationships are vital for maintaining optimum health. In fact, not feeling connected is as bad for us as obesity and smoking.

Humans have an inbuilt need to feel connected; it seems that our friends really do have a beneficial effect on our health:

- Close social contact helps to lower blood pressure and overall risk of heart disease.
- Women without a strong social and emotional support network are nine times more likely to develop a malignant breast tumour.
- Loneliness and social isolation are major risk factors for emotional conditions ranging from depression and anxiety to Alzheimer's disease, and can also cause sleep problems.

Friends for life

A large analysis of data from 148 studies involving more than 300,000 men and women found that those with poor social connections were 50 per cent more likely to die during the follow-up period of seven and a half years than those with good social ties. The boost in longevity was similar to the mortality difference between smokers and non-smokers and larger than that seen for many other lifestyle factors, including lack of exercise and obesity. And it didn't seem to matter whether the friends were male or female, or how old they were.

Interestingly, however, friends seem to be more important than even close relatives. One ten-year study of almost 1,500 people aged seventy and above found that a network of good friends was more likely to increase longevity in older people than close family relationships. While close contact with children and other relatives had little effect on longevity, those with lots of good friends and confidants lived, on average, 22 per cent longer than those with few friends. That's the difference between living to a hundred and dying at the age of seventy-eight. Surprisingly, these positive benefits persisted despite other profound life events such as the death of a spouse or another close relative. Of course, this doesn't mean that relatives aren't important to older people – only that they do not appear to influence survival.

Why friends count

No one knows for sure why friends are so important, as lonely people do not seem to be susceptible to any one disease in particular. Overall, it's thought that lonely people are more likely to rely on unhealthy coping mechanisms such as smoking, excessive drinking and over-eating. They are also less motivated to exercise on their own, and more prone to stress, as they have no one to confide in during difficult times. Stress increases blood pressure and heart rate, lowers immunity and leads to fatigue, as well as accelerating the ageing process.

In contrast, close friends might encourage older people to take greater care of themselves, to avoid smoking and drinking, and to seek medical advice sooner rather than later, when health problems arise. But caring relatives are likely to do just the same, so it's obviously more complicated than that.

DID YOU KNOW?

Talking to someone for just 10 minutes a day helps to improve your memory and mental performance. Socializing is as effective at sharpening the mind as more intellectual tasks such as reading-comprehension exercises and completing a crossword.

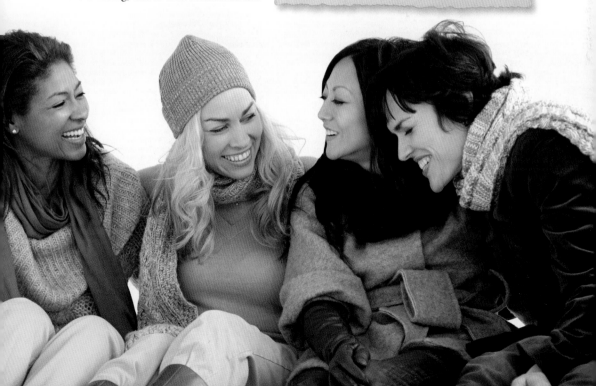

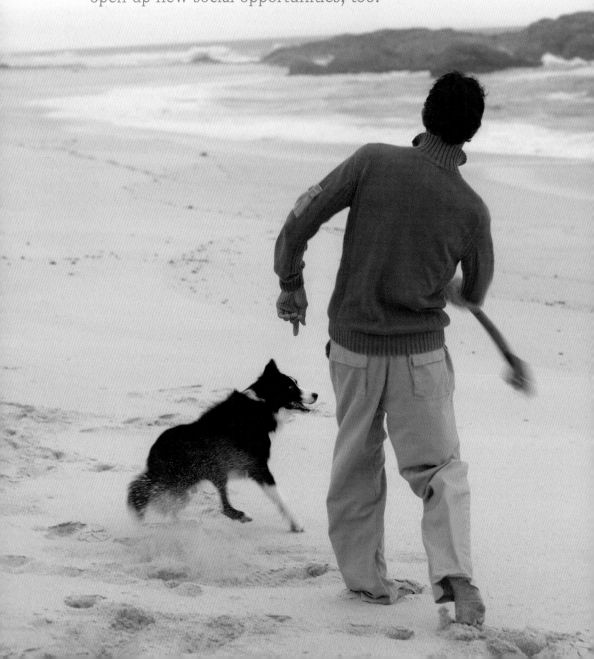

Keeping a pet is good for your health, and can open up new social opportunities, too.

SOCIAL SUPPORT

Studies suggest that, in a stressful situation, your blood pressure and heart rate increase less when you are accompanied by a person who is close to you. Brain imaging also shows a different pattern of brain activity when you're not alone during stressful times. In addition, people who are exposed to cold viruses are less likely to develop symptoms the more social connections they have, as frequent contact with other people helps to prime immunity.

The link between longevity and friends may even result from effects on self-esteem and the will to live. Whatever the cause, don't ignore your friends, and actively cultivate new ones throughout your future lifespan.

Feeling close to others is as vital for your health as getting your five-a-day and hitting the gym, so aim to prioritize time with your nearest and dearest. If you feel lonely, take steps to get out and meet new people with similar interests. Explore new hobbies or join an evening class to expand your skills. Or look into volunteering opportunities with local charities and community projects; it's a great way to meet others and feel as though you're making a difference.

Pet power

Keeping a pet is of great benefit for those who live alone, as well as being good for our health in general. Stroking a pet releases the feel-good hormone oxytocin. It also gives you a purpose,

LIVE HAPPY

Happy people live longer than depressed people. Scientists have found that asking yourself, every day, how happy you are on a scale of 1 to 10 produces valid results. If the value is less than 5, give yourself a treat to lift your happiness level.

so that – no matter how low you feel – you still have to get up to feed your pet and, if it's a dog, take it for exercise. This opens up new social opportunities, as dog walkers tend to strike up conversations with each other, helping you feel connected to people, too.

According to the Canine Charter for human health, drawn up by Dogs Trust, the UK's largest dog welfare charity:

- dog owners make fewer visits to their doctor
- owning a dog can help reduce blood pressure, stress and anxiety
- owners who walk their dogs are healthier than non-dog owners
- dogs can help the development of children with autism and children with learning difficulties
- owning a dog can boost your immune system
- dog owners are likely to recover quicker from heart attacks
- dogs can help safeguard against depression
- trained dogs can detect a variety of health conditions – including epileptic fits, cancerous tumours and hypoglycemia

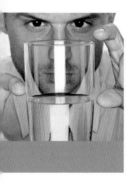

16 THINK positively

A positive outlook and optimistic view of ageing has been shown to influence how long we live. Surprising as it may seem, smiling through adversity can add more years to your life than not smoking.

Everyone ages, but how successfully we do so depends on our positivity. A study involving 660 people suggests that those with positive perceptions of their own ageing, and who view the ageing process optimistically, live, on average, seven and a half years longer than those who hate growing older. And this effect remained, regardless of other factors such as actual age, gender, income, loneliness and general health status.

Interestingly, this study compared the death rates of participants to the answers they gave to a survey twenty-three years previously. This suggests that adjusting your perception of ageing while you're still young has a significant effect on your life expectancy. So, look forward to those wrinkles – and you'll get longer to enjoy them.

MAPPING MOODS

Researchers from Cornell University in the US monitored 2.4 million users on Twitter, the online social networking service, in eighty-four countries over a two-year period, to assess the world's mood swings. They found that people mostly wake up in a good mood but this soon deteriorates once the work day begins. During the week, our happiest tweets are early in the morning and again near midnight. At weekends, the morning 'happy' peak occurs around two hours later in the day – presumably after a lie-in.

Where there's a will ...

Precisely why optimism promotes longevity remains unknown. Researchers believe that staying positive about growing older has a direct impact on our will to live, and ensures we remain proactive about our health – for instance, following a healthy diet, exercising regularly and attending regular health screenings. And, taking steps to follow a healthy diet and lifestyle pays dividends, as:

- **maintaining a low blood pressure,** by reducing salt and taking any prescribed medications diligently, can add four years to your life

- **maintaining low cholesterol levels,** through healthy diet and taking any prescribed statin drugs religiously, can add another four years to your life
- **watching your figure** and maintaining a healthy weight can add one to three years to your life
- **regular exercise** can add another one to three years to your life

A positive attitude also appears to reduce mental stress, improve resilience, and has favourable effects on immunity and brain function.

Believe in yourself

Positive thinking in the form of self-belief also contributes to a longer, more productive lifespan. Those who believe they can learn from their mistakes have different brain reactions to those who think it's not worth trying harder after a failure.

In a recent experiment, psychologists measured brainwaves in volunteers as they performed a task in which it was easy to make a mistake – identifying the middle letter of a series such as MMMMM or MMNMM. When participants made a mistake, their brain tracings showed an initial 'Oh crap' response as they realized their error, followed milliseconds later by a second response that showed whether they were likely to right the wrong. Those who believed they could learn from their mistakes had a stronger second response, and went on to pay more attention and do better, than those who believed intelligence is fixed and that there's little point in trying to change things. This form of self-belief is associated with age-related wisdom and a happier, positive view of the ageing process.

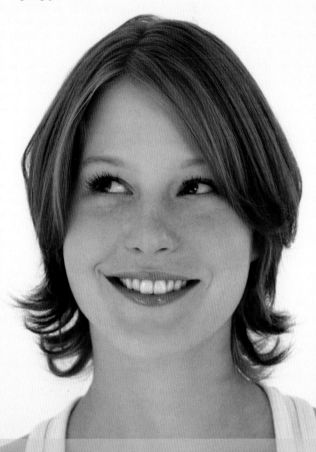

Smiling through adversity can add years to your life.

Laugh out loud

Laughter also has a beneficial effect, to the extent that humour is as good for you as a healthy diet and aerobic exercise – especially if you're prone to heart disease.

When you have a good laugh, your blood vessels dilate, supplying more oxygen-rich blood to your heart muscle. In contrast, when you feel stressed, your coronary arteries constrict. How did scientists make this discovery? By showing volunteers extracts from the comedy movie *There's Something About Mary* or distressing scenes from the epic war drama *Saving Private Ryan*. Blood-vessel diameter varied from 30 to 50 per cent, depending on which movie clips were shown to volunteers – and the reversal occurred within minutes.

Monitoring your emotions

Keep a mood log for a few days to score your own emotional well-being, using the points system outlined below. If your positive emotions are outweighed by the negative ones, aim to find more reasons to smile, laugh, feel happy and enjoy interesting pursuits. Listen to others and treat them with respect, so they are likely to do the same for you.

If you recognize that a particular negative emotion, such as stress, anger, sadness or worry, dominates your thoughts, you may benefit from counselling.

Add 1 point for every time in the day that you:
- smile or laugh
- are treated with respect
- feel enjoyment
- feel happy
- learn or do something interesting

Subtract 1 point for every time you experience:
- worry
- sadness
- anger
- stress
- depression

Meditation

Meditation is a relaxation technique that promotes positive affirmations and helps us to distance ourselves from negative thoughts. New findings suggest that people who meditate regularly have more grey matter in certain parts of their brain than those who don't. The white-matter connections between these brain regions are also stronger, and electrical signals are processed more rapidly. As a result, the brains of those who meditate are more able to resist the normal shrinkage that comes with age.

This may indicate that meditation helps to slow the brain-ageing process, but it is also possible that people who inherit these brain characteristics are naturally drawn towards meditation. But if there's even a slim chance that meditation gives the brain a mental push-up, it's worth getting reacquainted with your yoga mat.

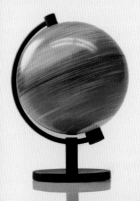

World Database of Happiness

Could where you live make a difference? The Erasmus University in Rotterdam has developed the World Database of Happiness based on scientific research into 'the subjective appreciation of life' in almost 100 countries. The happiest countries, according to how much nationals enjoy their life as a whole on a scale of 0 to 10, are as follows (*see* table below left; statistics based on 2009 data).

Although this does not necessarily equate to longevity, there is significant overlap with populations with the longest life expectancy (*see* highlighted countries), calculated in a recent study published in *The Lancet*, to suggest that our level of happiness may increase our lifespan. Both men and women living in Iceland, Sweden, Switzerland and Australia are among the happiest and longest-lived nationals in the world.

	COUNTRY	SCORE OUT OF 10
1	COSTA RICA	8.5
2	DENMARK	8.3
3	ICELAND	8.2
4=	SWITZERLAND	8.0
4=	CANADA	8.0
6=	FINLAND	7.9
6=	MEXICO	7.9
6=	NORWAY	7.9
9=	SWEDEN	7.8
9=	PANAMA	7.8
11=	AUSTRALIA	7.7
11=	AUSTRIA	7.7
11=	COLUMBIA	7.7
11=	LUXEMBOURG	7.7
15=	DOMINICAN REPUBLIC	7.6
15=	THE NETHERLANDS	7.6
15=	IRELAND	7.6

	LONGEST MALE LIFE EXPECTANCY	LONGEST FEMALE LIFE EXPECTANCY
1	ICELAND	CYPRUS
2	SWEDEN	SOUTH KOREA
3	MALTA	JAPAN
4	THE NETHERLANDS	GREECE
5	SWITZERLAND	ITALY
6	AUSTRALIA	SPAIN
7	NORWAY	SWITZERLAND
8	ITALY	AUSTRALIA
9	QATAR	SWEDEN
10	ISRAEL	ICELAND

HOW IT WORKS

Meditation involves focusing the mind to control physical and emotional symptoms and to achieve a state of calm and heightened awareness. Those experienced in meditation can quickly enter a trance-like state in which the brain generates special theta waves associated with creativity, visions and profound relaxation. People who mediate have higher levels of melatonin, nature's sleep-enhancing hormone, which is why meditation has been shown to improve sleep quality. It also reduces pain perception in people with fibromyalgia.

● **Mindfulness meditation** is one of the most popular forms, as it encourages you to focus on the present moment. You pay close attention to everyday activities such as preparing food or walking, concentrating on the sensations, textures, colours, smells and sounds involved. This prevents your mind spinning off and dwelling on potentially negative thoughts. It has been used to reduce stress, lower blood pressure, lift mood and reduce pain. It also has beneficial effects on immunity.

In one study, twenty-five people were vaccinated with flu vaccine after an eight-week course of mindfulness meditation, and the results compared with a group who had not meditated. Researchers found significant increases in antibody responses to the vaccine; brainwave patterns during the meditation course showed a beneficial activation of the front, left side of the brain, and the size of this activation was linked with the antibody response. This suggests that a short programme in mindfulness meditation produces beneficial effects on both brain and immune function, especially valuable as you get older.

● **Transcendental Meditation** (TM) is suitable for those who prefer a more structured approach, and is practised twice a day, for 20 minutes per sitting. TM uses the silent repetition of

EXERCISE: MINDFULNESS OF BREATHING

This exercise allows you to become aware that you are breathing, and of how you feel while you are breathing.

- Sit comfortably and close your eyes.
- Take a few long, slow deep breaths in and out.
- As you breathe out, let go and relax, as you focus your attention on the present moment.
- Then, let your breathing return to normal and 'watch' each breath as it is.

Find a place within your body where you feel the sensation of breathing most clearly, and let your attention rest there as you breathe normally. When your mind wanders, relax and let your mind experience the sensations of breathing again. When you feel ready, open your eyes, stretch and enjoy the sense of calm that flows through you.

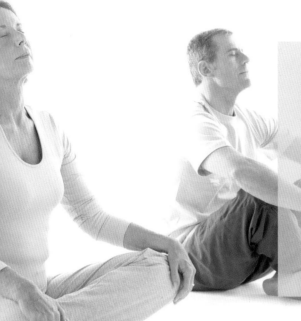

Sanskrit mantras (short words or phrases) to still your thoughts and body, so you achieve a state of restful alertness. *Relaxation response meditation* is a Westernized form which uses the principles of TM without the Eastern spiritual context. Relaxation exercises are combined with Western phrases – instead of Sanskrit mantras, you choose words that are rooted in your own belief system, such as 'calm' or 'peace'.

EFFECT ON LONGEVITY

Meditation-induced changes in state of consciousness are widely believed to extend human life and reverse age-related decline. To test this, seventy-three residents living in eight homes for the elderly (with an average age of eighty-one) were randomly assigned to either no treatment or one of three programmes teaching TM, mindfulness meditation

or relaxation. The results showed that improvements in cognitive flexibility, learning, word fluency, mental health, systolic blood pressure and behavioural flexibility were greatest in those learning TM and mindfulness meditation.

After three years, 100 per cent of those practising TM and 87.5 per cent of those performing mindfulness meditation were still alive, compared with 63 per cent of the remaining population. This suggests that meditation has positive effects against the ageing process and can prevent or even reverse decline in functioning that otherwise tends to occur among the elderly – even when started late in life. The meditation groups also reported that they felt better able to cope, less old and less impatient than before – which brings us back to the power of positive thinking with regard to the ageing process.

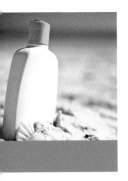

17 TAKE SOME sun

Sunscreen is vital to protect against skin cancer and the ageing effects of sunlight, but it also reduces the production of vitamin D in your skin, so you need to take steps to ensure you're still getting enough of this essential vitamin.

Our skin is one of the first parts of the body to show visible signs of ageing. The main external cause of fine lines and wrinkles is exposure to sunlight; both UVB and UVA are responsible. Most UVB is absorbed in the outer epidermal layer of the skin, while UVA penetrates more deeply to damage both the epidermis and dermis. As UVA rays can pass through glass, this means you're also exposed even when you're in a car, for instance, or sitting by an office window.

When ultraviolet light strikes the skin, it generates free radicals, which set up an inflammatory reaction known as heliodermatitis. This damages skin structures and interferes with normal cell division to increase the risk of skin cancer. Enzymes released during this process also damage elastin and collagen fibres, which provide structural support. In addition, natural substances in the skin that attract and trap water slowly disappear. The overall result? Skin loses its resilience and elasticity, to develop wrinkles.

DID YOU KNOW?

Studies by the American Academy of Dermatology reveal that, by the time you're eighteen, you have already received half your lifetime's quota of sun damage – much of it while playing outdoors as a child.

Sensible sun exposure

We produce much-needed vitamin D_3 when ultraviolet light interacts with a cholesterol-like substance in the skin ... but we also need to apply sunscreen to protect against the effects of UV radiation. In order to balance adequate production of vitamin D against the risks of skin cancer associated with excess sun exposure, the best advice is to obtain 10–15 minutes of sun exposure – without sunscreen – to the face, arms, hands or back, two or three times a week. Longer exposures don't provide additional benefit, as vitamin D is rapidly degraded by excess UV radiation.

For longer periods, when any part of your skin will be exposed to the sun for more than 20 minutes, use sunscreen. Apply it liberally (most of us don't use enough – it takes 25 g/1 oz to cover the entire adult body sufficiently) 15–30 minutes before exposure. And, unless otherwise instructed, reapply every two or three hours, and also after swimming.

SUNSCREEN PROTECTION

Sunscreens are rated according to their sun protection factor (SPF), which shows how effective they are at filtering UVB rays. Select a product with at least SPF15 (which absorbs 93 per cent of UVB rays) and preferably higher. For children, sunblock or an SPF of at least 30–40 is advisable.

CAUTION!

Take extra care when the UV index is particularly high, as unprotected skin will burn rapidly. Levels tend to be higher in the southern hemisphere, meaning that the risk of skin damage is greater.

For full protection, select products that screen out UVA rays too.

When used in the recommended quantities, sunscreen with a sun protection factor of 8 (SPF8) reduces vitamin D production in the skin by 95 per cent, while SPF15 reduces production by 99 per cent. The development of a tan when wearing sunscreen, however, suggests that, although you did not burn, enough UVB radiation reached the skin to

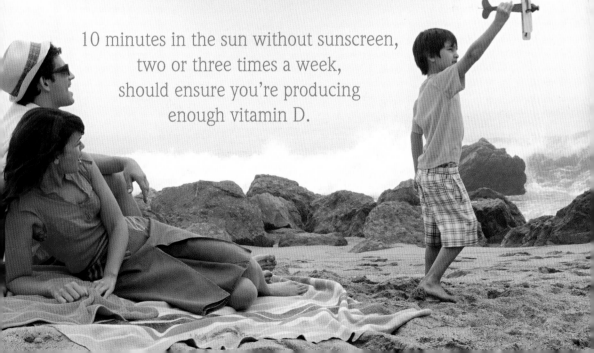

10 minutes in the sun without sunscreen, two or three times a week, should ensure you're producing enough vitamin D.

stimulate production of both melanin (a natural sunscreen produced in response to UV damage) and some vitamin D, regardless of sunscreen use.

Why we need vitamin D

Vitamin D has long been known to boost the absorption of calcium and phosphorus from the gut, but scientists are now discovering many more roles it plays in combating a number of common conditions that deteriorate with age.

Osteoporosis Vitamin D is important for calcium deposition in bone and for maintaining bone density. A large analysis of studies involving over 42,000 adults found that taking supplements of over 10 mcg (400 IU) vitamin D per day could reduce non-vertebral bone fractures by at least 20 per cent for individuals aged sixty-five and older.

Osteoarthritis Some studies have found a three- to four-fold increase in the risk of osteoarthritis progression in those with low vitamin D intakes, compared with people obtaining high intakes. One study involving eighty-two women and thirty-five men undergoing total hip or knee replacement found that 85 per cent had a vitamin D deficiency, compared with around 15 per cent of the general population.

Cancer Vitamin D binds to cell receptors to regulate gene activity and reduce abnormal cell growth. It has been shown to reduce growth and division of cancer cells in over 25,000 laboratory studies, and may help to protect against certain cancers, particularly those affecting the prostate, colon and breast.

Heart disease Vitamin D is involved in calcium metabolism and may help to reduce the amount of calcium laid down in artery walls as part of the hardening and furring-up process. It also has beneficial effects on blood pressure control. Studies suggest that people with the lowest vitamin D levels are 30 per cent more likely to have high blood pressure and 98 per cent more likely to have type 2 diabetes, which is another risk factor for heart disease. Overall, people with low vitamin D levels are twice as likely to experience a heart attack or stroke over a five-year period than those with higher levels – even when adjusting for other risk factors such as obesity and smoking.

Immunity Vitamin D boosts immune function to protect against infections. For example, research involving over

19,000 adults and adolescents found that those with the lowest vitamin D levels were 40 per cent more likely to develop a common cold. Those with low levels of vitamin D also appear to have a higher risk of developing asthma, and of being admitted to hospital with an asthma attack.

Brain health Scientists have recently discovered that vitamin D receptors are widely distributed throughout the brain, and appear to be directly involved in learning, memory and mood. Vitamin D may therefore have a protective role to play against dementia, Parkinson's disease and multiple sclerosis.

MAKE SURE YOU'RE GETTING ENOUGH

Where you live makes a difference. Our skin only produces vitamin D when the UV index is greater than 3, so there is a wide seasonal and regional variation in the amount produced by people in different countries. For example, those living at a latitude of 52 degrees north (which passes through the centre of the UK and Canada) are not exposed to enough UVB radiation to make vitamin D between October and April, while those living at 42 degrees north (the northern limit of Spain and part of the border between Canada and North America) are unable to synthesize vitamin D from November to February.

VITAMIN D SUPPLEMENTS

Some experts suggest that, during absences of exposure to sunlight, a minimum intake of 20 mcg (800 IU) is needed per day to maintain healthy blood levels of vitamin D during winter months. Others argue that intakes of 40 mcg (1600 IU) a day are needed, irrespective of sun exposure. Look for supplements providing vitamin D_3, as this appears to be 20–40 per cent more effective in maintaining blood vitamin D levels than the vitamin D_2 form.

A meta-analysis of data from eighteen clinical trials, involving over 57,000 people, found that those taking vitamin D supplements daily, with an average dose of around 13 mcg (528 IU), were 7 per cent less likely to die from any medical cause during the average follow-up period of almost six years.

Researchers have found that – with the exception of Norway, where intakes of vitamin-D-rich fish are high – most Europeans have low vitamin D levels during winter. Vitamin D levels are also low in those who habitually wear clothes that cover most of their skin, or who stay indoors most of the time.

As we age, our ability to produce vitamin D reduces; at the same time, there is evidence to suggest that our need for vitamin D increases. It is therefore important to select foods that are fortified with vitamin D, or to take a vitamin D supplement (*see* above).

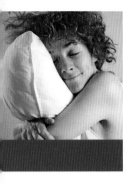

18 GET A GOOD
night's sleep

Sleep is when the body carries out repairs, and getting the right amount lowers blood pressure and reduces the risk of heart disease, as well as boosting your immunity and combating depression.

Sleep is a natural form of unconsciousness in which some parts of the brain switch off but others become more active. It is a time of profound relaxation that is so essential for our physical and mental well-being that we spend around a third of our lives in bed. While you are asleep:

- your brain processes information, memory and experiences
- your muscles and joints recover from constant use during the day
- you produce increased amounts of growth hormone
- protein in all parts of your body is replenished faster than when you are awake

- your production of skin cells, red blood cells and immune cells increases

Types of sleep

There are two main types of sleep:
- **Rapid Eye Movement** (REM) sleep, in which your eyes are constantly moving
- **Slow Wave** sleep, in which your eyes stay relatively still

Slow Wave sleep has four stages. When you first fall asleep, you rapidly pass down through the lighter stages 1 and 2, before spending 70–100 minutes in the deeper stages 3 and 4. Sleep then lightens again and a short period of around 10 minutes' REM follows. This cycle repeats four to six times throughout the night, but, as morning approaches, an increasing amount of time – up to one hour – is spent in REM sleep.

As you get older, you naturally spend less time in deep stage 4 sleep. By the age of seventy, many people get no stage 4 sleep at all.

DID YOU KNOW?

Although alcohol helps you fall asleep, you are likely to wake and have a disturbed night once the drug effect wears off. Try a warm milky drink instead!

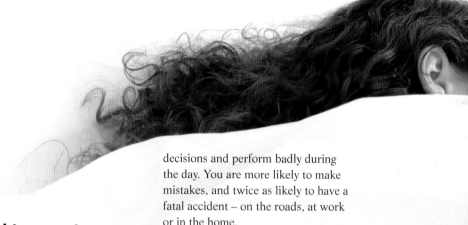

The right amount

Achieving just the right amount of sleep seems to be important for long-term good health. Studies have consistently shown that sleeping for 7–8 hours is associated with the lowest risk of chronic disease and adult age-related mortality.

Researchers who followed 21,000 sets of twins for over twenty-two years, for example, found that those who slept for between 7 and 8 hours per night lived longer than those who habitually slept for shorter or longer periods. And a recent study involving 1,700 adults also found that men who habitually slept for less than 6 hours were four times more likely to die during the fourteen-year duration of the study than those who slept for longer, even after taking other factors such as blood pressure and diabetes into account. Interestingly, however, the researchers did not find a link between mortality risk and insomnia or short sleep-duration in women in this study.

Accidents When you don't get enough sleep you wake up feeling tired and irritable, and tend to make poor

decisions and perform badly during the day. You are more likely to make mistakes, and twice as likely to have a fatal accident – on the roads, at work or in the home.

Heart disease Tiredness appears to increase the risk of developing high blood pressure. Compared to those with normal sleeping habits, those who sleep for less than 5 hours are five times more likely to develop hypertension, while those who sleep for 5–6 hours are three and a half times more likely to have high blood pressure. This effect is seen at any age, which means teenagers who sleep for less than 6½ hours a night are two and a half times more likely to have an elevated high blood pressure than those sleeping for longer.

Depression Lack of sleep affects brain function; people with insomnia tend to report higher levels of stress, anxiety and depression than those who regularly enjoy a good night's sleep. If disruption to sleep is severe, it can act as a trigger for suicidal behaviour.

Immunity People exposed to a common cold virus are three times more likely to develop symptoms if they get less than 7 hours' sleep a night than if they achieve 8 hours' sleep or more.

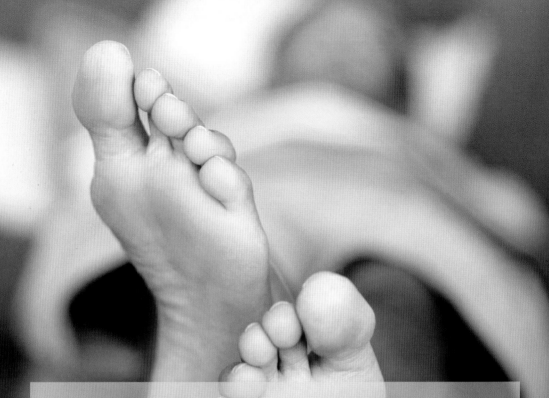

Tips for a good night's sleep

- **Avoid daytime naps,** which reduce your need for sleep at night.

- **Avoid over-indulgence** in substances that interfere with sleep, such as caffeine, nicotine and alcohol, and rich or heavy meals – especially in the evening.

- **Take regular exercise,** but avoid strenuous exercise late in the evening.

- **Take time to unwind** from the stresses of the day before going to bed; read a book, listen to soothing music or have a candlelit bath.

- **Don't take worries to bed with you.** If something is worrying you, write it down and promise yourself you will deal with it in the morning.

- **Learn to associate the bedroom with sleep** – don't use it for study, eating, working or watching TV.

- **Maintain a regular sleep routine,** going to bed and rising at the same time every day.

- **Make sure that your bedroom is dark and quiet,** and also a comfortable temperature and humidity.

- **Inhale lavender essential oil** for its soporific effects.

Obstructive sleep apnoea (OSA)

People who suffer from this common sleep-related breathing disorder literally stop breathing during sleep for 10–30 seconds at a time. This occurs when part of the upper airway collapses, blocking the inflow of oxygen to the lungs and the outflow of carbon dioxide. The commonest cause is over-relaxation of throat muscles, which allows the upper airway to sag or the tongue to fall backwards. This is especially likely in overweight people who store fat around their neck. Enlarged glands (tonsils, adenoids or thyroid) can also play a role.

The blocked airway usually results in loud snoring, followed – when complete obstruction occurs – by a cessation of breathing. Failure to breathe causes carbon dioxide to build up in the blood, which activates a survival mechanism in the brain to restart the breathing process. As the airway is jerked open again, a gasp occurs and the sufferer may briefly wake up. These episodes can lead to significant daytime sleepiness if they last for more than 10 seconds each time and occur more than ten times a night.

The severity of OSA is classified according to the number of times per night you stop breathing or experience significantly reduced air flow. Research suggests that those with moderate to severe OSA, who experience fifteen or more episodes per hour, have an increased mortality risk (of dying from any cause) of up to six times, compared with those who don't have OSA – so it's in your long-term health interests to try and treat it.

> ## DID YOU KNOW?
>
> **Playing the** didgeridoo has been shown to improve snoring and sleep apnoea by strengthening throat muscles in the upper airway.

OVERCOMING OSA

If you suffer from OSA, here are some tips to help beat it:

- lose any excess weight
- stop smoking
- take regular exercise
- use anti-snoring devices and sprays
- raise the head of your bed 10 cm (4 in) to help stop your tongue flopping back
- try wearing dental appliances at night to stop the tongue falling back or to lift the soft palate to keep the airway open
- continuous positive airway pressure (CPAP) delivered at night via a mask can also keep the airway open
- in some countries, the stimulant drug modafinil is licensed to treat excessive sleepiness in people with OSA

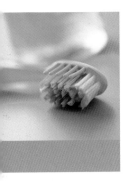

19 FLOSS YOUR teeth

It's estimated that daily flossing can add over six years to your life. Why? Because it reduces gum disease, which has now been identified as a risk factor for coronary heart disease as well as other conditions.

The mortality rate for people with inflamed gums (gingivitis, periodontitis) is up to 46 per cent greater than for those with healthy mouths. Inflamed gums allow mouth bacteria to enter the circulation, especially if they bleed during brushing. Until recently the link between gum disease and heart disease was based on observations that those with gum disease are twice as likely to develop coronary heart disease and three times more likely to have a stroke. Those with the highest level of periodontal bacteria (in the gum pockets around the teeth) also have

a higher risk of developing blockages in the carotid arteries of the neck and, for men, of experiencing erectile dysfunction. Some evidence also suggests that inflammatory chemicals entering the circulation from inflamed gums may worsen insulin resistance and glucose control, to increase the risk of type 2 diabetes.

Arterial plaque and gum disease

As you get older, the lining of your arteries naturally accumulates a build-up of fatty material called plaque. This thickens, may accumulate calcium, and can eventually cause significant hardening and narrowing of the arteries in a process called atherosclerosis.

A number of factors promote the progression of fatty deposits in your artery walls, causing them to become more extensive. These include all the usual suspects, such as family history, smoking, obesity, lack of exercise, an unhealthy high-fat diet, lack of dietary antioxidants, high blood pressure,

FIGHT THE FAT WITH FLOSS

Fatty arterial streaks are present in 20 per cent of children aged two to fifteen years, 60 per cent of young adults aged twenty-six years, and 70 per cent of those aged forty. By the ages of fifty and over, they are almost universal. So, the earlier in life you start flossing, the better!

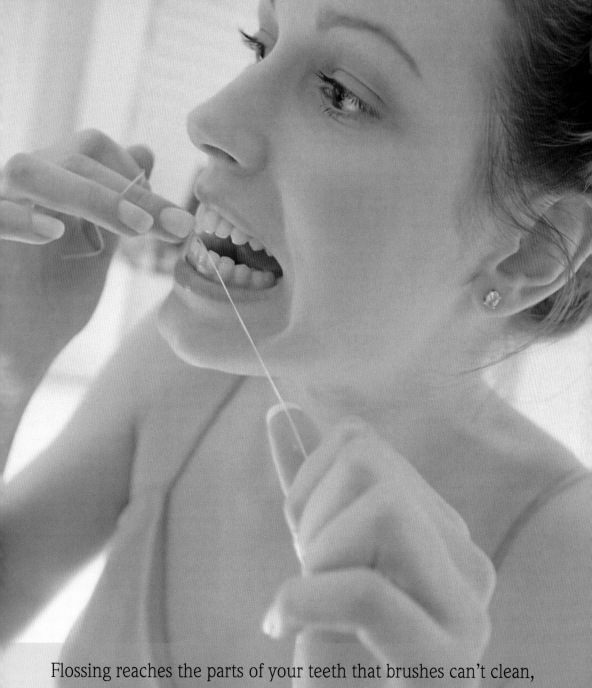

Flossing reaches the parts of your teeth that brushes can't clean,
helping you to minimize the risk of gum disease.

raised cholesterol levels, raised triglyceride levels and poor glucose control. However, these classic risk factors only explain about half of the observed features of cardiovascular disease, and gum disease has now joined the list of possible missing links.

MOUTH BACTERIA

Researchers from the University of Florida have now found live mouth bacteria within artery-clogging plaque to prove the connection. The bacteria found include *Porphyromonas gingivalis* and *Actinobacillus actinomycetemcomitans*, which are leading causes of periodontal disease and adult tooth loss, plus species of *Veillonella*, *Chryseomonas* and *Streptococcus*. Those with the highest level of these bacteria in their mouths also had a correspondingly high level in their arterial plaque. The level of white blood cells found within the arterial plaque is also linked to the number of bacteria present. This suggests that,

in some cases, heart disease could be classed as an infectious disease, with the arterial damage resulting from the immune response your body mounts against the bacteria detected within artery walls.

Hanging by a thread

Your lifespan could be hanging by the proverbial thread – in the form of dental floss! Regular flossing reaches the parts of your teeth that brushes can't clean, to remove decaying food particles and mouth bacteria.

A wide range of flossing products are available, including:

- **Standard floss:** varieties include thin, expandable, silk, woven, waxed, mint-flavoured
- **Flossers:** short strands of floss pre-loaded onto a disposable handle
- **Floss picks:** less damaging than toothpicks and make access to difficult areas easier
- **Interdental brushes:** tiny brush-like flossing devices (available in different sizes) that gently ease into the space between teeth without forcing
- **Floss threaders:** ease flossing in tight or obstructed areas (for use with bridges, braces, crowns and implants)
- **Water jets:** a less fiddly alternative to flossing and, as well as being easier to use, twice as effective as string floss for reducing gum bleeding and improving oral health. Water flossing claims to remove 99.9 per cent of plaque

Could antibiotics prevent heart disease?

New research raises the intriguing possibility that antibiotic treatment might protect against coronary heart disease – partly by killing the mouth bacteria present in plaque, and partly by protecting against a common respiratory infection, *Chlamydia pneumoniae*, which is also linked with heart attack. People with high antibody levels against *Chlamydia pneumoniae* have over double the risk of a heart attack, compared to those with low levels. And, in smokers, the risk is almost doubled again, even when other risk factors such as family history, high blood pressure, raised cholesterol levels and diabetes are taken into account. Studies suggest that 50–60 per cent of patients suffering a heart attack have high antibody levels to *C. pneumoniae*, compared with only 7–12 per cent of healthy adults.

Unfortunately, these mouth and respiratory bacteria are widespread. Most of us will experience at least one *Chlamydia pneumoniae* infection during our lifetime. Seven out of ten people develop no symptoms, while others suffer relatively mild problems such as sore throat, cough, sinusitis or laryngitis. In those who are particularly susceptible, it can cause more serious lung diseases such as pneumonia or bronchitis.

If your immune system successfully clears these infections, there is no long-term problem. Sadly, *Chlamydia* bacteria have an unpleasant tendency to hang around in the body, causing chronic (long-term) infections, and have also been identified in arterial plaques.

KEEP ON FLOSSING

If these bacterial links to heart disease are proven, it raises the interesting possibility that a prolonged, tailored course of antibiotic treatment could prevent a future heart attack in a significant number of people. Trials using standard antibiotics, however, have so far proved unsuccessful, as the bacteria are safely tucked away inside the fatty plaques where antibiotics cannot penetrate. So – for the time being – flossing remains your best protection.

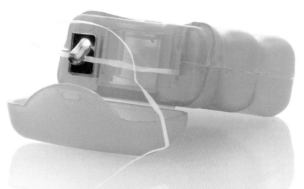

Regular flossing may even help protect against heart disease.

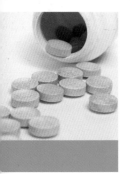

20 CONSIDER
supplements

Although you can age gracefully on your own, certain supplements do offer anti-ageing benefits that can potentially slow the process down, should you decide to give yourself a helping hand ...

There is such a wide variety of supplements now available that it can be difficult to know where to start. Here are some of the most beneficial general anti-ageing supplements on offer, with recommended daily doses listed for each. Select the ones most suited to your needs or, alternatively, try the combination suggested on page 105, if you're still unsure which way to go. (Advice on supplements to target specific body areas is included in the Body Tour section in Part Two.)

● **Multivitamin and mineral supplements** guard against nutritional deficiencies that have adverse effects on metabolism (for example, B vitamins)

and immune function (such as vitamin D). While diet should always come first, several studies have found that people who take a multivitamin and mineral supplement are less likely to develop cold symptoms than those not taking supplements – and this is particularly true for older people. One study found that those taking a multivitamin supplement for one year experienced half as many days ill with infections as those not taking multivitamin supplements.

A scientific review of over 150 clinical trials, published by the American Medical Association, showed that nutrient deficiencies are a key risk factor for heart disease, stroke, some cancers, osteoporosis, and other age-related, major health problems, with the authors going as far as to state that 'it appears prudent for all adults to take vitamin supplements'.

Daily dose: Select one designed for your age group (for example, 50+, 70+) or one providing 100 per cent of the recommended daily amount (RDA) for as many vitamins and minerals as possible

CAUTION!

If you are pregnant, taking any prescribed medication or are in any way concerned about taking supplements, seek advice from your doctor first.

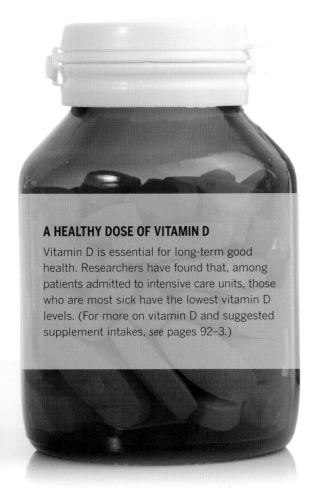
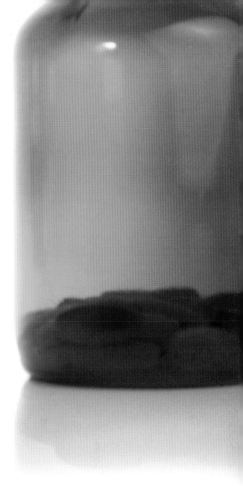

A HEALTHY DOSE OF VITAMIN D

Vitamin D is essential for long-term good health. Researchers have found that, among patients admitted to intensive care units, those who are most sick have the lowest vitamin D levels. (For more on vitamin D and suggested supplement intakes, *see* pages 92–3.)

● **Antioxidants** reduce the number of ageing oxidation reactions to which your cells are exposed. Researchers from the Human Nutrition Research Center on Aging at Tufts University, Massachusetts, calculate that we each need 3,000 to 5,000 ORAC units per day to achieve good tissue antioxidant levels. The average person eating three portions of fruit and vegetables per day only achieves a daily intake of 1,200 ORAC units, giving a shortfall of between 1,800 and 3,800 units on a daily basis. This shortfall can be made up by taking antioxidant supplements (for more information on ORAC *see* Eat More Fruit, page 16):

Vitamin C: Humans are one of the few animals unable to synthesize their own supplies. As a result, some scientists claim this genetic accident means we all suffer from a hereditary disease, hypoascorbaemia, which increases our risk of viral infections, raised cholesterol levels, coronary heart disease and cancer, as well as reducing our ability to cope with the effects of stress. **Daily dose:** 250–1000 mg

Vitamin E: A study of over 11,000 people aged sixty-seven years plus found those taking vitamin E supplements had a one-third lower risk of death, at any age, compared with those not taking them. A review of over a dozen studies involving centenarians also showed that those who survive into their 100s have exceptionally high blood levels of vitamin E compared with those found in younger adults. Always combine with other antioxidants (especially vitamin C), which regenerate it and prolong its effects. **Daily dose:** 12–540 mg

Selenium: This provides one of your most important antioxidant defences against cancer. Supplements have been shown to reduce the risk of cancer-related deaths by over 50 per cent – in fact, one medical trial was stopped early, as it was considered unethical to withhold selenium from those taking inactive placebo. **Daily dose:** 200 mcg

Carotenoids: Lutein and zeaxanthin protect against age-related macular degeneration (one of the most common causes of visual loss in later life), while tomato lycopene protects against atherosclerosis and some cancers, especially those of the prostate gland. **Daily dose:** 6 mg mixed carotenoids

● **Alpha-lipoic acid** (ALA) works together with B-group vitamins to speed energy production in cells. It boosts the uptake of glucose into muscle cells, which improves glucose control, and helps to reduce glucose uptake into fat cells, to slow middle-age spread. ALA also helps to protect the nervous system from the effects of ageing by reducing the breakdown of the fatty sheath surrounding nerve fibres. In addition, it may reduce the progression of some forms of dementia.
Daily dose: 50–100 mg

● **L-Carnitine** helps to mobilize fat stores and regulate energy production. It may play a useful role in reducing middle-aged spread and has beneficial effects on cholesterol and triglyceride levels. It also improves fatigue.
Daily dose: 500 mg – 3 g, usually in divided doses

● **Co-enzyme Q10** is vital for energy production in cells, especially contracting heart muscle cells. After the age of twenty, levels of CoQ10 decrease, as less dietary CoQ10 is absorbed and its production in body cells declines. Low levels of CoQ10 mean cells do not receive all the energy they need and are more likely to become diseased and age prematurely. Declining levels of CoQ10 therefore contribute to the ageing process, including coronary heart disease and heart failure.
Daily dose: 100–200 mg (higher dose essential for those taking a statin drug to lower cholesterol levels, as statins switch off CoQ10 production in the liver)

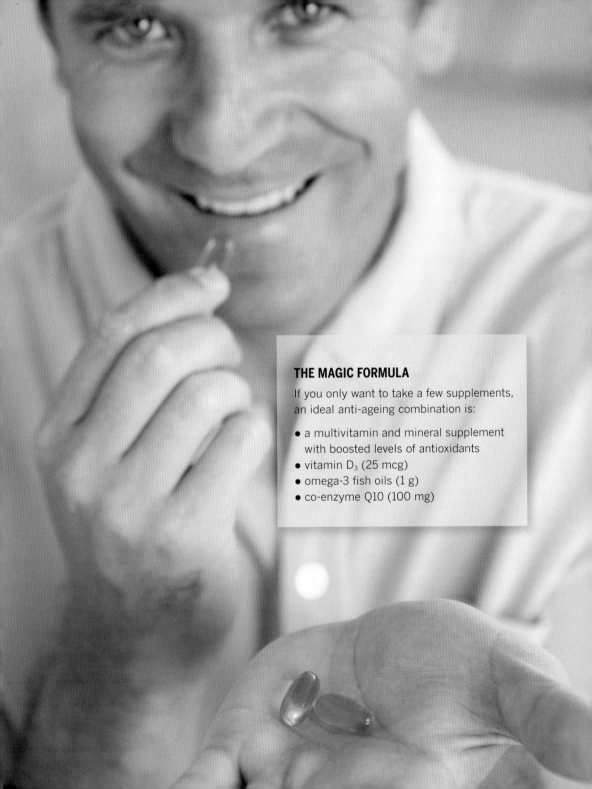

THE MAGIC FORMULA

If you only want to take a few supplements, an ideal anti-ageing combination is:

- a multivitamin and mineral supplement with boosted levels of antioxidants
- vitamin D₃ (25 mcg)
- omega-3 fish oils (1 g)
- co-enzyme Q10 (100 mg)

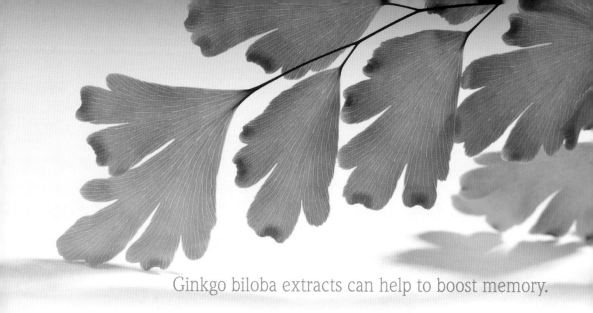

Ginkgo biloba extracts can help to boost memory.

● **Folic acid** lowers levels of homocysteine – an amino acid that damages artery linings when allowed to build up in the circulation. High homocysteine levels are linked with many conditions, including dementia, heart disease and stroke. Those with the highest intakes are 45 per cent less likely to experience a heart attack than those with the lowest levels. Folic acid works best when combined with vitamins B_6 and B_{12}, which lower homocysteine in a different way.
Daily dose: 400–800 mcg

● **Garlic** has beneficial effects on blood pressure, blood stickiness, cholesterol balance and arterial elasticity to reduce the risk of heart attack by at least 30 per cent. It also boosts immunity against infection and has powerful anti-cancer effects: a meta-analysis of results from eighteen studies suggests that those consuming the most garlic (more than 28.8 g/1 oz garlic per week) were 31 per cent less likely to develop colorectal cancer, and 47 per cent less likely to develop stomach cancer, than those consuming the least. (*See also* Eat More Garlic, pages 30–33.)
Daily dose: 600–900 mg standardized garlic powder tablets

● **Ginkgo biloba** provides unique antioxidants that improve blood flow to the peripheries, including the brain. This helps to boost memory in some older people and may show benefits against dementia. It is also helpful for people with poor circulation in the fingers and toes, and may offer some benefit for men with erectile dysfunction.
Daily dose: 120–240 mg

● **Ginseng** is one of the oldest known herbal medicines, used as a revitalizing and life-enhancing tonic for over 3,000 years. Traditionally, ginseng is described

as stimulant, restorative and energizing, helping to improve immunity, strength, stamina and alertness. It contains an enzyme, panquilon, which appears to have a similar action to that of the anti-impotence drug sildenafil.
Daily dose: 200–600 mg

• **Glucosamine** promotes the formation of new cartilage and has anti-inflammatory actions to reduce pain in ageing joints. It is often taken together with chondroitin, which works together with glucosamine to inhibit the breakdown of cartilage. Glucosamine is one of the most important supplements for people over the age of fifty, when joints start to cause symptoms of creaking, pain stiffness, knobbiness and reduced mobility.
Daily dose: glucosamine 1500 mg / chondroitin 1200 mg

• **Isoflavones** Researchers suggest that soy isoflavones could have the potential to prolong life. They have been found to activate an anti-ageing protein, Sirt-1, that protects our DNA and is involved in the regulation of ageing and longevity (*see also* Eat More Beans, page 26). This may partly explain the long life expectancy and healthy ageing observed in the inhabitants of Okinawa Island in Japan, who also practise dietary restriction (*see* Eat More Vegetables and Eat Less Overall, pages 22 and 62). Isoflavones are also beneficial for menopausal symptoms in women.
Daily dose: 40–100 mg

• **Omega-3 fish oils** have an anti-ageing effect throughout the body, especially the heart, circulation, brain and joints, and improve joint pain, stiffness and swelling. An intake of at least 1 g omega-3 fish oils per day (from eating oily fish twice a week, or from pharmaceutical-grade supplements) almost halves the risk of sudden cardiac death and helps prevent death due to coronary thrombosis (heart attack). Populations consuming the most fish also have the lowest level of sudden death from abnormal heart rhythms, stroke and depression. (*See also* Eat More Oily Fish, pages 40–45.)
Daily dose: 1 g

• **Plant sterols** block the absorption of dietary cholesterol to lower levels of harmful LDL-cholesterol by around 15 per cent. This significantly reduces the risk of experiencing heart disease or stroke.
Daily dose: 1–3 g

• **Reishi** Known as the 'mushroom of immortality', it is traditionally used to strengthen the liver, lungs, heart and immune system, to increase intellectual capacity and memory, boost physical and mental energy levels and to promote vitality and longevity. Research suggests it boosts immunity, lowers blood pressure and reduces fatigue and the harmful effects of stress.
Daily dose: 500 mg twice or three times daily

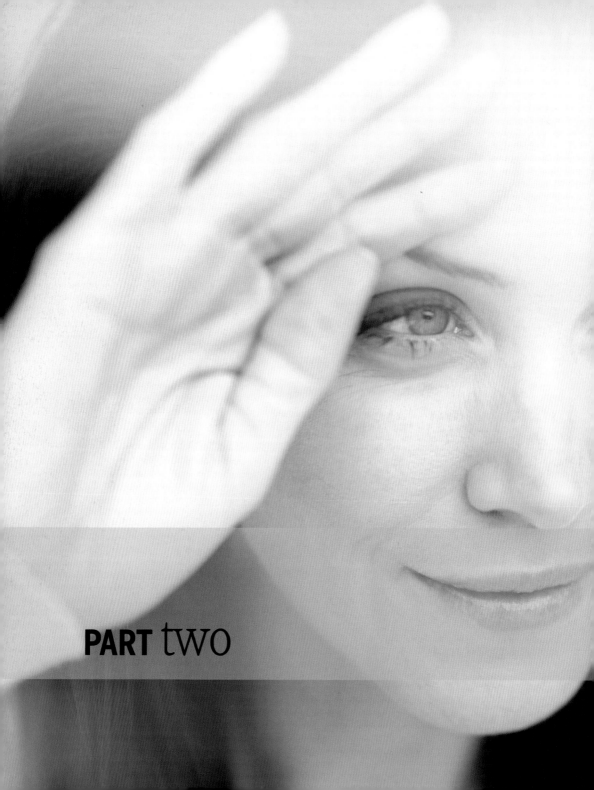

PART *two*

body TOUR

Check out how specific body parts and functions age,
and what you can do to minimize the effects.

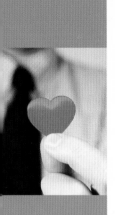

Heart

Your heart contracts and relaxes around seventy times a minute, 100,800 times per day and over 2.76 billion times during an average lifespan to keep blood flowing round your body. And, if you look after it, it can beat for significantly longer!

COMMON PROBLEMS

Because heart muscle contracts regularly, it needs a ready supply of oxygen, glucose and other nutrients. If this supply fails, due to narrowed or blocked arteries, you will experience heart-muscle pain known as angina. If the blood supply to your heart is compromised more severely – for example, by a blood clot or arterial spasm – then a heart attack occurs, as heart-muscle cells die.

Other age-related problems include heart failure, when weakened muscle no longer pumps efficiently, and valvular heart disease, in which damaged heart valves either fail to open properly (known as stenosis) or fail to close properly (known as incompetence), or both. Valvular heart disease affects blood flow so that excess fluid pools in the ankles (causing swelling), lungs (causing breathlessness), or both.

Looking after your heart

Failure to pay attention to your diet and lifestyle may result in your heart failing prematurely, too. Most heart problems are linked with an unhealthy diet containing too many processed foods and excess refined carbohydrates (especially sugar and white flour), and not enough wholegrains, fruit and vegetables. Concentrate on obtaining wholefoods and beneficial fats such as fish, olive, rapeseed and walnut oils, while cutting back on processed foods such as doughnuts, cakes and biscuits. Eat at least five servings of fruit and vegetables daily, and cultivate a love – if you don't already have one! – for the humble yet antioxidant-rich cup of tea (*see* pages 58–61).

Medical **ALERT!**

Chest pain or discomfort should always be taken seriously and medical advice sought without delay. Chewing an aspirin can be life-saving in the case of a heart attack, as it helps to break up newly formed blood clots.

You can also reduce your risk of heart disease by:

- **Not smoking** – smokers are five times more likely to have a heart attack in their thirties and forties than non-smokers, and three times more likely to have one overall.
- **Losing any excess weight**, especially the 'menopot' (abdominal fat forming a 'pot belly', often present in post-menopausal women).
- **Exercising regularly** for at least 30 minutes, on most days.
- **Limiting your alcohol intake** to remain within recommended safe guidelines.
- **Cutting back on salt intake** – don't add salt during cooking or at the table, and compare labels to select products with the lowest content of salt/sodium chloride.
- **Avoiding excess stress**, which increases your blood pressure by an amount equivalent to carrying an extra 20 kg (44 lb) in weight, or an additional twenty years in age.

Anti-ageing supplements

Fish oils *have a thinning effect on the blood, lower blood pressure and reduce abnormal heartbeat rhythms; if you suffer from heart disease, it can reduce your risk of a fatal heart attack by a third*

Garlic tablets *improve arterial elasticity and blood flow*

Folic acid, vitamin B$_{12}$ *and* **vitamin B$_6$** *help to lower levels of homocysteine, an amino acid that can hasten narrowing of the arteries*

Plant sterols *effectively lower a raised cholesterol level*

Co-enzyme Q10 *for energy production in heart-muscle cells (especially important for those taking a statin drug to lower cholesterol, to help avoid statin side effects such as muscle aches and fatigue)*

Isoflavones *help to boost oestrogen levels in post-menopausal women and have a protective effect on arterial elasticity*

- **Knowing your blood pressure** and cholesterol levels, so that you are aware of any changes.
- **Maintaining tight control of risk factors** for heart disease, such as high blood pressure, diabetes and raised cholesterol (through diet, lifestyle and any necessary prescribed medication).

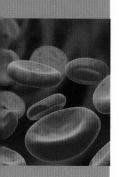

Circulation

Your circulation transports oxygen and nutrients around your body, as well as carrying away waste products for excretion, so it's vital to do as much as you can to keep it working smoothly.

Arteries carry blood away from the heart and have thick, elastic walls to carry pulsating blood under high pressure. Large arteries branch and divide into a series of narrower arterioles, which, in turn, connect to capillaries – tiny vessels with thin walls that allow oxygen, nutrients, fluid and wastes to pass to and from your tissues. Capillaries are connected to small veins called venules, which feed into larger veins that carry blood back to the heart.

ATHEROSCLEROSIS

Atherosclerosis – hardening and furring-up of the arteries – is strongly linked with increasing age, smoking, lack of exercise and eating an unhealthy diet containing too much fat and too few antioxidants (fruit and vegetables). It is more likely to occur in those who have uncorrected high blood cholesterol levels, high blood pressure and poorly controlled diabetes, so it's essential to ensure these are all well controlled.

VARICOSE VEINS

The long veins in the legs contain a series of valves that allow blood to flow upwards against the pull of gravity. Weak valves frequently give way due to backward pressure, so that blood pools in the veins just under the skin, which become dilated and twisted. This can cause aching and dragging sensations, swelling of the ankles and feet, itching, bleeding and phlebitis – inflammation of a superficial vein due to clotting of poorly circulating blood.

QUICK FACTS

- The circulatory system contains 150,000 km (90,000 miles) of blood vessels
- Your circulation contains around 5 litres (5.3 quarts) of blood
- The heart pumps the equivalent of 13,640 litres (14,410 quarts) of blood per day
- Blood flows through the main arteries at a rate of 1.2 m (4 ft) per second
- Blood flows through the great veins at an average rate of 10 cm (4 in) per second

Avoid standing for prolonged periods of time, as this encourages blood to pool in the legs. When sitting, put your feet up as much as possible to help reduce blood pooling in your lower limbs. Support stockings or tights will help to keep varicose veins comfortable – have them correctly fitted by a pharmacist.

Looking after your circulation

As well as following a generally healthy a diet, try to:

- **Cut back on salt** – this can lower blood pressure and reduce the rate of atherosclerosis. Avoid obviously salty foods (such as crisps, bacon, pickled fish/meats, products tinned in brine) and stop adding salt during cooking or at the table.
- **Avoid getting too cold**, as this causes small blood vessels to go into spasm, reducing blood flow to peripheries, especially fingers and toes. This can lead to chilblains (itchy, purple areas of inflammation) and Raynaud's syndrome, in which small arteries in

the fingers and toes constrict. Fingers initially go white, with numbness and tingling; as sluggish blood flow returns, the digits go blue, then bright red with pain and burning. Keep extremities warm during cold weather with gloves, hat, scarf, thick socks and ankle warmers.

- **Take regular exercise**, especially walking, as contraction of leg muscles boosts blood flow through your lower limbs by up to a third.

Anti-ageing supplements

Antioxidants *help to lower blood pressure and reduce atherosclerosis*

Omega-3 fish oils *have a blood-thinning effect that can improve peripheral circulation*

Folic acid *helps to lower blood levels of homocysteine, an amino acid which can damage artery linings (vitamins B_{12} and B_6 also have a beneficial effect)*

Ginkgo biloba *and* **garlic extracts** *can improve general circulation to the peripheries*

Pycnogenol *and* **red vine leaf extract** *can both improve venous circulation and reduce ankle swelling*

Co-enzyme Q10 *increases oxygen uptake in cells and may reduce the pain associated with poor circulation*

Calcium *and/or* **magnesium** *supplements may reduce muscle cramping*

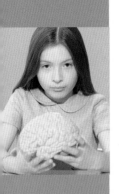

Brain

Your memory is a personal storehouse of information but, as we age, facts become harder to store and retrieve. There's no shame in using notes to jog your memory, but there are ways to enhance your recall, and give your brain a helping hand ...

The brain contains over a hundred billion brain cells, or neurons, that are found in the outer, folded grey matter. These receive and interpret sensory information, co-ordinate muscle contraction and perform all the processes involved in thinking, speaking, writing, singing, calculating, creating, planning and organizing.

But, sooner or later, most of us will begin to experience 'senior moments' – those temporary lapses in memory when you can't recall someone's name, for instance, or remember what it was you meant to do when you left the room.

The good news is that you *can* take steps to do something about it. In fact, it's estimated that the risk of dementia can be as much as halved through simple diet and lifestyle changes.

Looking after your brain

- **Exercise regularly** to increase blood flow to the brain, supplying oxygen and nutrients. In one study, those who walked, on average, one mile per day, developed less shrinkage of their grey matter over a nine-year period than those who were sedentary, and were half as likely to experience muddled thinking.
- **Avoid smoking cigarettes** – and, if you do smoke, quit. Smoking causes spasm of blood vessels and hastens hardening and furring-up of the arteries, reducing blood flow to the brain.
- **Eat more fruit and vegetables** – these contain vitamins, minerals, antioxidant polyphenols and other substances that help to lower blood pressure. And, those with low blood pressure during middle age are four to five times less likely to develop dementia due to the arterial damage associated with hypertension. If

Medical ALERT!

If memory loss is accompanied by confusion, poor concentration or a change in behaviour or personality, it's important to seek medical advice.

Anti-ageing supplements

Folic acid and **vitamin B$_{12}$** *lower levels of homocysteine – an amino acid that can hasten narrowing of the arteries to worsen memory loss*

Vitamin D *is directly involved in learning, memory and mood, and may have a protective role against dementia*

Ginkgo biloba *improves blood flow to the brain and may protect short-term working memory*

Omega-3 fish oils *have blood-thinning effect to improve blood flow and protect against depression*

Phosphatidylserine *boosts synthesis of brain chemicals and helps to improve cognitive functions, including learning, recall, recognition and concentration*

Isoflavones *have been shown to help boost memory in older women*

Pine bark extracts *improve circulation to the brain and may improve memory and ability to think straight*

your BP is raised, take medication to control it (check with your doctor).

- **Eat more fish**, especially oily fish, as the omega-3 fish oils they contain play an important structural and functional role in the brain. People who eat fish or seafood at least once a week have a lower risk of developing dementia and depression. Fish oils also protect against stroke.
- **Avoid excessive alcohol**, as this impairs some aspects of auditory and visual memory and your ability to remember word sequences.
- **Get a good night's sleep** – some types of spatial memory (for example, finding your way around) are only laid down if learning is followed by a period of sleep. Those who complain of poor sleep appear to be more at risk of dementia.
- **Learn a new skill** – when it comes to brain power, it's a case of 'use it or lose it'! Keep your mind active to increase the connections between brain cells and reduce pruning of those that aren't used. Solve crosswords or Sudoku puzzles, or try tackling other types of brain-training puzzle. Join the free online Scrabble site (www.isc.ro) and play people from all over the world at any time of day or night.
- **Avoid middle-age spread** – becoming obese, especially during middle age, doubles your risk of dementia, especially if you tend to store excess weight around your waist.

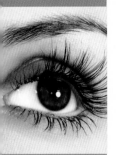

Eyes

Often referred to as the windows of the soul, your eyes provide a good visual clue to how well you are ageing – inside and out. A number of conditions can affect the eyes as you get older, but dietary and lifestyle changes can help.

COMMON AGE-RELATED CONDITIONS

Dry eyes, due to reduced tear production, become more common with increasing age, but also watch out for the following:

Cataracts are opacities in the normally crystal-clear eye lens that occur when lens proteins undergo changes similar to those that turn cooked egg white from clear to cloudy. This results in blurring, sensitivity to sun glare, changes in colour perception, and seeing haloes around light. Most cataracts are due to degenerative changes with increasing age, and are worsened by exposure to ultraviolet light.

Age-related macular degeneration (AMD) is a painless, progressive loss of central vision which causes visual distortion, typically obliterating words when you try to read, and blanking out someone's face when you look straight at them. AMD is associated with reduced levels of carotenoid pigments in the macula – a part of the retina responsible for fine vision. These yellow pigments, lutein and zeaxanthin, filter out harmful blue light and neutralize the damaging chemicals produced during light detection.

Glaucoma develops when fluid pressure in the eye increases enough to compress the small blood vessels that nourish the optic nerve, and may lead to loss of vision.

IT'S ONLY NATURAL

Presbyopia is a form of long-sightedness that is a normal part of the ageing process. Your eye lens continues to grow throughout adult life, while the eye stays a fixed size. The lenses also thicken and become less elastic, so it is increasingly difficult to focus on near objects. Symptoms start appearing around the age of forty-five, so that corrective lenses are needed for close activities such as reading. Visit an optician if you notice a change in your eyesight.

Looking after your eyes

Eyes that are clear, vibrant and sparkling appear more youthful than dull, tired eyes surrounded by bags and crow's feet – so do your best to achieve the former! Similar diet and lifestyle changes help to protect against each of these age-related problems.

- **Get a good intake of dietary antioxidants** from fruit and vegetables – aim for at least five servings per day, and preferably more. Those that are most protective for eyes include lutein-rich kale, spinach, broccoli and orange-yellow sweetcorn, peppers, apricots and mangoes, as well as dark berries.
- **Eat at least two servings of oily fish per week** – omega-3 fish oils play an important structural and functional role in the retina at the back of the eye.
- **Wear sunglasses** that carry the UV400 mark to protect your eyes from the sun.
- **If you're a smoker, quit** – smokers are three times more likely to develop cataracts and four times more likely to experience AMD than non-smokers.
- **If you use a computer, take frequent breaks** to reduce the chance of eye strain and tiredness. Look away from the screen during 'thinking time' and focus on objects at varying distances away. Remember to blink to reduce dry-eye problems.
- **Have regular eye check-ups,** at least once a year.

Anti-ageing supplements

Antioxidant vitamins A, C, E *and the mineral* **selenium** *protect the eye against the damaging effects of light*

Lutein *and* **zeaxanthin** *('nature's sunglasses') are especially protective against AMD*

Omega-3 fish oils *help to maintain optimum visual perception in the retina and brain*

Bilberry extracts *contain anthocyanin blue-red pigments that protect against AMD, cataracts and diabetic retinopathy*

Pine bark extracts *can reduce the progression of retinopathy and improve visual acuity in people with diabetes*

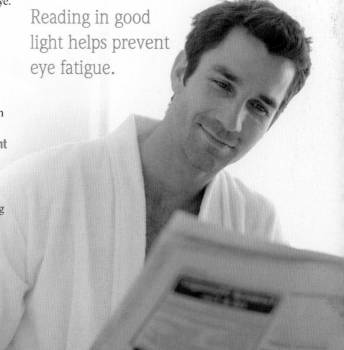

Reading in good light helps prevent eye fatigue.

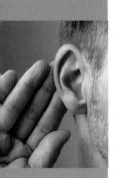

Hearing

Loss of hearing becomes an increasingly common problem with age, and can have a variety of causes, depending on the part of the ear affected. Dietary factors can help.

Your ears are divided into three parts – the outer, middle and inner ears. The outer ears collect sound vibrations and funnel them through the external auditory canal to the tympanic membrane, or eardrum. Movement of this membrane triggers a chain of movement in three tiny bones within the middle ear. These hinged bones, called ossicles, amplify the vibrations and pass them on to the inner ear. Here, the vibrations stimulate hair-like cells, each of which responds best to a single frequency. These hair cells send electrical impulses to the brain, which are interpreted as sound.

QUICK FACTS
- Humans can normally distinguish over 400,000 different sounds
- The hearing range for a young adult is 20 to 20,000 Hz
- The hearing range in an older person decreases to around 50 to 8,000 Hz

HARD OF HEARING?
A number of age-related problems can reduce hearing:

Earwax can build up to block sound transmission. While soft wax naturally makes its way out of the ear canal, wax tends to become more profuse with age.

Presbycusis is an age-related hearing loss caused by deterioration of vibration-sensitive hair cells in the inner ear. It affects one in two people over the age of seventy-five and tends to creep up slowly, reducing your ability to hear high-frequency sounds, such as 's', 'sh', 'th' and female voices.

Otosclerosis is another cause of age-related hearing loss, in which the tiny bones in the middle ear fail to pass on sound waves properly to the inner ear.

Looking after your ears
- **Try to keep your ears dry**, if you are prone to wax build-up. Wax absorbs water and swells to make symptoms worse. Semi-hard earwax

can often be dislodged by oily ear drops inserted at night. Plug the ear with cotton wool to prevent staining of your pillowcase. Drops that 'fizz' can help to dislodge more stubborn wax (ask your pharmacist for advice). Otherwise, ear syringing can be performed by a healthcare professional.

- **Increase your intake of carotenoid-rich vegetables** (green leaves and orange vegetables such as sweet potatoes). People with the highest intakes, in addition to vitamin-E-rich foods such as almonds, appear to have a reduced risk of moderate or greater hearing loss, compared with those who have the lowest average intakes of these nutrients.

Anti-ageing supplements

Antioxidants *such as vitamins C and E may help to preserve hair cells in the inner ear*

Omega-3 fish oils *may be beneficial for those who eat little oily fish*

Ginkgo biloba extracts *may help to reduce tinnitus (ringing in the ears)*

- **Eat two servings of oily fish per week**, such as salmon, and you will be significantly less likely to experience hearing loss than those who eat less fish.
- **Visit a hearing-aid specialist**, if your hearing is becoming impaired – ask your doctor for a referral. Modern hearing aids are small and sophisticated, helping to filter out or augment different sounds levels to improve clarity of hearing. Many opticians now supply hearing aids as well as spectacles.

CAUTION!

Never attempt to clean your ear by inserting an object such as a cotton bud or swab. This will push the wax plug further down, may damage the eardrum and can even dislocate the tiny bones in the middle ear to cause permanent deafness.

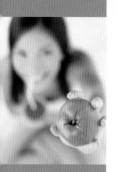

Taste AND smell

The scent and flavour of different foods adds greatly to our quality of life. Most of us notice these pleasures dwindling as we get older, however – but is there anything we can do about it?

HOW WE TASTE

Our taste receptors are located on small bumps on the surface of the tongue, called papillae. These have a central pore, filled with saliva, into which dip tiny sensory nerve endings which detect dissolved chemicals. When stimulated, these receptors send messages to the brain to detect different flavours. Six different taste perceptions – bitter, sweet, salty, sour, savouriness and 'fatness' – combine to produce an overall taste sensation. Other nuances of flavour come from your senses of smell, texture, temperature, astringency, spiciness, coolness (for instance, menthol), numbness, fizziness, metallic taste and mouth feel (known by the Japanese term *kokumi*), with additional input from visual and auditory stimuli.

As we age, we lose taste receptors, so fewer are present, and those that remain also become less sensitive. And the same is probably true for olfactory receptors …

HOW WE SMELL

When we inhale, aromatic chemicals are drawn up towards smell receptors at the top of the nose. Aromatic molecules, known as odorants, dissolve in mucus overlying the olfactory epithelium (specialized membranous tissue inside the nasal cavity). They are detected by tiny, hair-like sensory nerve endings (cilia) that project from the dendrites (branched extensions) of olfactory receptor cells into the overlying mucus. Odorants bind to specific receptors on the cilia, each of which only detects one particular smell. You have an estimated 12 million olfactory receptor cells, which are divided into around 1,000 different odorant-receptor types. Each type only responds to a specific group of odorant molecules. These receptors are directly wired into the brain, and pass messages to the emotional centres of the limbic system to evoke powerful emotional responses, including those associated with fear, love and sexual attraction.

The average person can detect 4,000 different odours, but whose with a gifted 'nose' can detect as many as 10,000 different smells.

Looking after your senses

Lack of zinc is one of the most common causes of age-related loss of sense of taste (ageusia) and sense

Anti-ageing supplements

Zinc *is best taken in a supplement that also provides potassium, magnesium, calcium and vitamin B$_{12}$, which are important for smell/taste sensation; it is also usually taken with copper to balance copper metabolism*

Curcumin *(extracted from turmeric) has powerful anti-inflammatory actions that may improve loss of taste and smell associated with rhinitis (nasal inflammation)*

N-acetylcysteine, *an amino acid, makes mucus less viscous and may improve symptoms by alleviating mucus blocking sense receptors*

Testing for zinc deficiency

Zinc deficiency can be tested for by obtaining a solution of zinc sulphate (15 mg/5 ml) from a pharmacist. Swirl a teaspoonful in your mouth:

- if the solution seems tasteless, zinc deficiency is likely
- if the solution tastes furry, of minerals or slightly sweet, zinc levels are borderline
- if the solution tastes strongly unpleasant, zinc levels are normal

of smell (anosmia). This most often results from a poor diet. Sources of zinc include red meat, seafood (especially oysters), offal, brewer's yeast, wholegrains (although processing removes most of their mineral zinc), pulses, eggs and cheese.

Do what you can to improve your dietary intake, but it's a good idea to take a zinc supplement, too (*see* above).

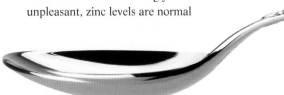

Zinc can help boost your sense of taste and smell.

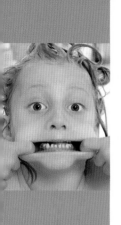

Teeth AND gums

Healthy gums and teeth are so important for youthfulness that being 'long in the tooth' is considered a sign of old age. But many people in the prime of life are also affected, as receding gums are a common result of gum disease.

LACK OF SALIVA

Saliva keeps gums healthy by washing the mouth clean and providing antibodies and other substances that reduce bacterial infection. It also contains enzymes that break down food trapped between the teeth, and minerals that help to neutralize the acids produced by plaque bacteria. Saliva production often falls with increasing age, however, and lack of saliva leads to decay and loss of dental enamel at the base of the teeth.

If your mouth feels dry, use an artificial saliva spray and chew sugarless lozenges or gum, which, as well as stimulating saliva production, contain xylitol – an artificial sweetener that protects against dental decay.

ACIDIC-FOOD DAMAGE

Tooth enamel readily dissolves on contact with acid substances with a pH (measure of acidity) of less than 5.5. Once dissolved, enamel can't be recovered, and the softer, underlying parts of the tooth soon decay.

The acidity of many common foods and drinks is surprisingly high; the substances listed below, for example, can all harm your teeth with prolonged contact.

FOOD/DRINK	PH
LEMON/LIME JUICE	1.8–2.4
BLACK COFFEE	2.4–3.3
VINEGAR	2.4–3.4
FIZZY COLA DRINKS	2.7
ORANGE JUICE	2.8–4.0
APPLES	2.9–3.5
GRAPES	3.3–4.5
TOMATOES	3.7–4.7
MAYONNAISE/SALAD DRESSING	3.8–4.0
BLACK TEA	4.2

Try to select fruit juices fortified with added calcium, as this decreases their erosive potential. If you are consuming fizzy or acidic drinks, drink them quickly and use a straw (positioned towards the back of your mouth) to lessen the contact time between your teeth and the drink.

TEETH-GRINDING

One in twelve people grind their teeth while asleep, and one in five clench their jaws while awake. Bruxism (grinding) weakens your teeth, and can lead to tension headache and aching jaws, too. You could be a grinder if:

- your teeth look worn down, flattened or chipped
- you develop increased tooth sensitivity, or wake with jaw pain, tightness in jaw muscles, earache, a dull headache
- you have chewed tissue on the inside of your cheeks

Once teeth are worn away, the damage is permanent, so prevention is key. Your dentist can fit a soft plastic mouthguard designed to prevent teeth damage (to stop grinding, a more expensive hard, acrylic mouthguard is needed). Cutting back on alcohol and caffeine intake and tackling causes of stress can also help, as can relaxation techniques such as yoga and meditation.

Anti-ageing supplements

Multivitamin and mineral supplements *protect against nutritional deficiency and improve gum health*

Co-enzyme Q10 *can reduce gum inflammation and help promote regrowth*

Calcium *improves the protective benefits of saliva, and may reduce bone-thinning in the jaw (leading to loosened teeth)*

Vitamin C *for collagen production in healthy gums*

Valerian *can reduce stress, improve sleep and may help with bruxism*

Looking after your mouth

- **Rehydrate your mouth regularly** by sipping water, and sluice your mouth out after drinking tea, coffee, cola, sports drinks and alcohol.
- **Rinse your mouth** with water rather than brushing immediately after eating. Abrasion from a toothbrush after consuming acidic drink/food may increase loss of enamel.
- **Have regular dental check-ups** (ask advice about using fluoride products, a soft toothbrush and low-abrasive toothpaste; dentists are also well placed to detect mouth cancers, whose incidence is rising).
- **Use toothpastes that contain antacids,** such as bicarbonate of soda, or sodium hexametaphosphate – a whitening ingredient which leaves a protective layer on teeth.

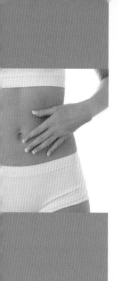

Gut

When your gut works properly, it's easy to take it for granted. But, as it's around 4 metres (13 feet) long, that means there's plenty of room for problems to occur ...

As you age, changing bowel function reduces secretion of intestinal juices (causing indigestion and bloating), slows transit time (leading to constipation) and affects bacterial balance in the large bowel, which can be associated with constipation, wind and discomfort. Reduced absorption of vitamins and minerals can also lead to nutritional deficiencies, especially of B vitamins and co-enzyme Q10, contributing to fatigue.

DYSPEPSIA

Dyspepsia (indigestion) becomes more common with increasing age, and includes any discomfort after eating, such as feelings of distension, flatulence, nausea, heartburn and acidity. This may be linked with acid reflux and reduced secretion of intestinal juices, including bile.

If you suffer from dyspepsia, steer clear of hot, acidic, spicy and pastry foods, which can lead to indigestion, and avoid heavy meals (especially in the evening). Instead, eat little and often throughout the day, rather than having three large meals. Cut back on alcohol intake and drink other fluids in small amounts at frequent intervals, rather than consuming large quantities at a time. Also avoid tea, coffee and acidic fruit juices if these trigger symptoms.

Losing any excess weight will also help to reduce reflux. Don't stoop, bend or lie down immediately after eating, and wear loose clothing,

Medical **ALERT!**

- If you suffer from recurrent indigestion or heartburn, or notice any persistent change in bowel habit, tell your doctor.
- If you regularly take antacids, speak to your doctor – one in ten regular users, especially those over the age of forty, could have a more serious underlying problem which needs investigation and treatment. Some bowel conditions, including bowel tumours, produce small amounts of hidden blood in the motions, which can be screened for.

The bowels contain 11 trillion bacteria, weighing a total of 1.5 kg (3¼ lb). Ideally, at least 70 per cent of these should be healthy probiotic bacteria and only 30 per cent other less beneficial bacteria, such as *E. coli*. In practice, however, the balance is usually the other way round.

Anti-ageing supplements

Ginger *helps to relieve indigestion and nausea*

Probiotics *replenish levels of beneficial bowel bacteria*

Globe artichoke *stimulates bile production and can reduce feelings of bloating and other symptoms associated with irritable bowel syndrome (abdominal pain, flatulence, constipation)*

Aloe vera *has a soothing antacid and analgesic action*

Psyllium seed and husks *are an effective, natural fibre source*

especially around the waist. If reflux and heartburn are a problem when lying down, try elevating the head of your bed 15–20 cm (6–8 inches) by putting books under the top two legs (make sure it's stable!).

Looking after your gut

- **Maintain plenty of 'friendly' bacteria.** Probiotic bowel bacteria play an important role in intestinal health. They ferment and break down undigested fibre and bulk up the stools to make defecation easier. The most important intestinal bacteria are those that secrete lactic acid. These are known as probiotic bacteria (such as *Lactobacilli* and *Bifidobacteria*) and help to promote good digestion, boost immunity and increase resistance to infection. To maintain a high population of probiotic bacteria in your intestines, consume live bio yogurts or probiotic drinks daily – select those containing

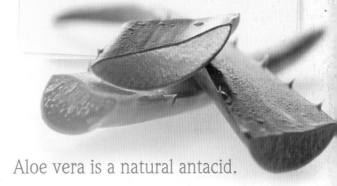

Aloe vera is a natural antacid.

clinically proven strains, such as Activia, Yakult and Actimel (also known as DanActive).

- **Make sure you're getting enough fibre.** To obtain the recommended 18–30 g (around ¾–1 oz) per day, eat plenty of fruit and vegetables – at least five servings a day, if you can. As well as providing bulk to promote bowel movements, fibre acts like a sponge, absorbing toxins and excess fats.

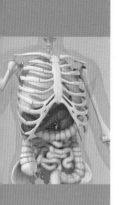

Liver

A healthy liver is a prerequisite for a long and healthy life, yet many people take their liver for granted. Following a healthy diet and lifestyle is the best way you can protect it.

Your liver sits in your upper-right abdomen, immediately below the diaphragm, and extends across above the stomach and pancreas. It is one of the most active and vital organs in the body, and also one of the most forgiving. Everything absorbed from your gut travels straight to your liver, where it is processed and detoxified. These processes generate inflammatory substances (free radicals and leukotrienes), and exposure to excess toxins can damage liver cells during the detoxification process.

Yet even when challenged by a fatty diet and regular exposure to toxins such as alcohol, its incredible powers of regeneration help it to struggle on. Even if a surgeon removes 75 per cent of a liver lobe, it usually tries to grow back.

WHAT YOUR LIVER DOES
- makes bile to aid digestion and emulsify dietary fats
- makes new body proteins, including those involved in clotting
- converts ammonia (a toxic waste product of protein metabolism) into urea
- processes dietary fats to make cholesterol and triglycerides
- helps to maintain blood sugar levels by manufacturing glucose
- stores excess glucose as glycogen (a starchy emergency fuel) to maintain blood sugar levels when needed (for example, during the overnight fast)
- stores fat-soluble vitamins (A, D, E and K) and some minerals (such as iron and copper)
- generates heat to warm passing blood
- helps to control blood-cell formation and destruction
- removes poisons (such as alcohol) from the blood and detoxifies them
- acts as an immune 'sieve', filtering out antigens absorbed via the intestines

In the long term, dietary over-indulgence (whether of calories, fats or alcohol) can lead to fatty degeneration. This produces liver changes similar to those seen in the force-fed duck and geese bred to produce *pâté de foie gras*. While this may be a culinary delicacy, doing the same to your own liver will compromise your chances of longevity. Fatty change can progress to liver inflammation (hepatitis), formation of scar tissue (fibrosis) or even cirrhosis – a serious condition in which the liver shrinks and becomes nodular.

Looking after your liver

- **Eat a healthy diet** supplying sufficient calories without excess, and plenty of fruit and vegetables for protective antioxidants.
- **Concentrate on obtaining healthy fats** (from olive, rapeseed, nut and fish oils), as these do not have a major impact on the amount of cholesterol manufactured in the liver.
- **Avoid excess alcohol**, as this is a cell poison that can cause inflammation and fibrosis of the liver in excess.
- **Avoid risky lifestyle activities** that increase your risk of exposure to hepatitis viruses that attack the liver and can cause long-term damage.

Anti-ageing supplements

Milk thistle seed extracts *help to boost levels of glutathione, a liver antioxidant that protects liver cells from toxic damage, making it useful for anyone who leads an excessive lifestyle*

Globe artichoke *has similar regenerating and protective properties to milk thistle. It stimulates liver function to increase bile production, lower cholesterol levels and improve 'bilious' symptoms (bloating, flatulence, nausea, abdominal discomfort)*

Probiotic bacteria (Lactobacilli, Bifidobacteria) *digest dietary fibre to produce short-chain fatty acids, such as propionate, which have an anti-inflammatory effect on the liver*

Probiotics *may also improve liver function by reducing gut 'leakiness' and the number of endotoxins absorbed into the circulation and taken to the liver for processing*

B group vitamins *for liver metabolism*

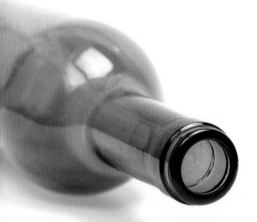

DID YOU **KNOW?**

Milk thistle helps to protect your liver before a heavy night out, while globe artichoke can reduce hangover effects the following morning (*see* supplements).

Avoid excess alcohol, to help keep your liver healthy.

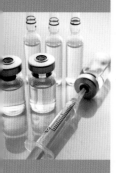

Pancreas

Following a low-GI diet will reduce your pancreas's workload, and also results in a number of other beneficial effects, including the improvement of risk factors for cardiovascular disease.

Your pancreas lies beneath the liver and has several important roles. As well as secreting powerful digestive enzymes that break down dietary proteins, fats and carbohydrates, it secretes hormones involved in glucose and appetite control. Important pancreatic hormones include:

- **glucagon** – raises blood glucose levels
- **insulin** – lowers blood glucose levels
- **amylin** – slows gastric emptying and digestion
- **somatostatin** – suppresses release of insulin and glucagon
- **ghrelin** – stimulates appetite by triggering feelings of hunger
- **pancreatic polypeptide** – released after eating to suppress appetite

FRUIT AND VEG

Most fruit and vegetables (excluding parsnips and potatoes) have a relatively low glycemic index/load and do not normally need to be restricted. Take care with dried fruit such as raisins, however, as the sugars are concentrated due to the evaporation of water.

DIABETES

Arguably the most important pancreatic hormone is insulin, which acts as the key to let glucose enter muscle and fat cells. Type 1 diabetes occurs when the pancreas stops making insulin – usually completely. This type is irreversible and treated with insulin injections. In contrast, type 2 diabetes occurs when you continue to produce some insulin, but not enough to control blood glucose levels properly. People with type 2 diabetes can often return to normal glucose control if they exercise regularly (to burn glucose), follow a low glycemic diet and lose excess weight.

Looking after your pancreas

LOW-GI DIET

Different foods have different effects on blood glucose levels, depending on the amount and type of carbohydrate they contain. Known as their glycemic index (GI), this is calculated by comparing how quickly the food raises glucose levels compared with glucose (which is assigned a standard GI of 100). Foods with a GI of 55 or less are classed as *low* GI, those with a GI of 56–69 are classed as *medium*, while 70 or above is classed as *high*. Typical GI values for common foods are shown below (GI values for other foods can be found at www.glycemicindex.com, courtesy of the University of Sydney).

	FOOD	GLYCEMIC INDEX
HIGH	Parsnips	97
	Baked potato	85
	Cornflakes	81
	Wholemeal bread	71
MEDIUM	Raisins	64
	White rice	64
	Porridge	58
	Wholemeal rye bread	58
	Muesli	56
LOW	Brown rice	55
	Honey	55
	Sweetcorn	54
	Kiwi fruit	53
	Banana	52
	Unsweetened orange juice	52
	Waxy new potatoes	50
	Mixed-grain bread	49
	Carrots	47
	White spaghetti	44
	Sweet potato	44
	Oranges	42
	Unsweetened apple juice	40
	Apples	38
	Wholemeal spaghetti	37
	Dried apricots	31
	Kidney beans	28
	Cashew nuts	22
	Raw cherries	22

Anti-ageing supplements

Chromium *is needed to make Glucose Tolerance Factor (GTF), which boosts insulin sensitivity*

Magnesium *is associated with insulin sensitivity and glucose tolerance; a diet rich in magnesium may even help to prevent the development of type 2 diabetes, especially in people who are overweight*

Zinc *for the synthesis, storage and secretion of insulin (some people with type 2 diabetes may have an inherited inability to transport sufficient zinc into pancreatic cells)*

Conjugated linoleic acid *helps to improve insulin sensitivity through its ability to mobilize and transport fatty acids away from fatty tissues to muscle cells, where they are burned for fuel*

You can reduce your insulin requirements, and improve glucose control in type 2 diabetes, by following a low-GI diet. This involves reducing your intake of high-GI foods, and selecting those with a low to moderate GI instead. You can also combine foods with a high GI (such as baked potatoes) with those that have a lower GI (such as beans) to help even out fluctuations in blood glucose levels.

As well as reducing your pancreas's workload, a low-GI diet helps you maintain a healthy weight, reduces the damaging effects of spiking glucose levels on your circulation, and has a favourable effect on other risk factors for cardiovascular disease, such as blood stickiness, blood pressure, triglyceride levels and cholesterol balance.

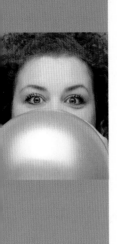

Lungs

Breathing is usually taken for granted, as it happens automatically – normally with little effort or thought. But many people develop poor breathing habits as they get older.

Deep sighing, gasping, breath-holding or rapid, shallow breathing can undermine well-being in several unexpected ways, by heightening the effects of stress, reducing oxygen perfusion of body tissues and possibly increasing your risk of high blood pressure, heart attack and stroke.

HYPERVENTILATION

When your breathing is shallow and rapid, you quickly blow off too much carbon dioxide, so your blood loses acidity and becomes more alkaline. This affects the transmission of nerve signals, causing symptoms of dizziness, faintness and pins and needles, often around the mouth. These symptoms heighten your sense of panic, making you breathe even faster, blowing off more carbon dioxide, and this can trigger a panic attack.

People who habitually hyperventilate sometimes experience a frightening number of other physical symptoms, including numbness, muscle spasm, chest pain, palpitations, visual disturbances, severe headache and even collapse.

OTHER PROBLEMS

Exposure to airborne pollutants, especially cigarette smoke, is the most common age-related challenge to the lungs. Inhaled pollutants lead to inflammation, with widespread stiffening, narrowing and airway obstruction. Inflammation also increases mucus production (chronic bronchitis), promotes lung infections (acute bronchitis, pneumonia) and can lead to the over-stretching and rupture of tiny air sacs (emphysema). Asthma can also develop in later life, due to abnormal immune responses that trigger airway inflammation and spasm with symptoms of cough, wheezing and shortness of breath.

CHECK YOUR BREATHING RATE

Ask a friend to count your breathing rate when you are unaware. The average breathing rate is ten to twelve breaths per minute, but people who hyperventilate regularly breathe at fifteen to twenty breaths per minute, and someone in a state of panic can reach as many as thirty breaths per minute.

Looking after your lungs

- **Practise calm breathing.** In the East, breathing lies at the core of meditation and yoga practices, which adepts believe can rejuvenate body and mind to promote health, strength and longevity. Imagine a candle just in front of your face, that flickers gently as you breathe in and out. Check your breathing pattern by placing one hand on your abdomen and the other on your upper chest; as you inhale, the lower hand should rise first.
- **Don't smoke,** and avoid smoky or polluted atmospheres.
- **Take regular exercise** but, if running or cycling on a regular basis, be sure to keep away from roads that expose you to heavy traffic fumes. Inhaling particles from diesel engines can increase the risk of heart disease as well as lung disease.
- **Drink coffee!** Coffee, dark chocolate and unsweetened cocoa are beneficial, as they contain methylxanthines such as caffeine and theobromine, which open up

Anti-ageing supplements

Antioxidants *such as vitamins C, E and pine bark extracts reduce inflammation*

Omega-3 fish oils *have a powerful anti-inflammatory action*

Turmeric *contains curcumin, which relaxes smooth muscles to reduce airway spasm*

Magnesium *inhibits constriction of airways and promotes their relaxation*

Co-enzyme Q10 *for oxygen utilization and energy production in cells (levels are reduced in those with lung disease)*

Reishi mushroom *has an immune-modulating effect to improve airway over-sensitivity*

the airways and reduce coughing. Regular coffee intake reduces the chance of wheezing by 30 per cent, compared with non-coffee drinkers. Ground coffee provides more benefit than instant coffee, but excess can cause tremor, sleep problems and withdrawal symptoms.

- **Eat a Mediterranean-style diet** providing plenty of antioxidant-rich fruit and vegetables and fish. Those who eat oily fish at least twice a week are half as likely to experience wheezing or chest tightness than those who eat little oily fish – even when other factors such as smoking are taken into account.

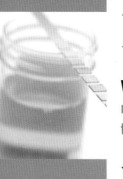

Kidneys

We tend not to give our kidneys much thought, but kidney function naturally reduces as we get older, and ageing kidneys can contribute to rising blood pressure, as well as other problems.

Your kidneys lie at the back of the abdomen, on either side of the spine. Each contains over a million filtration units, called nephrons. Blood flows into these filtration units under pressure, so that fluid and soluble substances such as urea are forced through the walls of small blood vessels into a collection system where some water, nutrients and salts are reabsorbed before excess trickles down to the bladder for storage.

NATURAL AGEING

The number of nephrons within the kidneys decreases from around the age of fifty onwards. This reduces their ability to filter water and salts, meaning that fluid retention may occur.

The kidneys also produce a hormone called renin. This activates mechanisms within the circulation that cause rapid constriction of arteries, so blood pressure increases. If arteries supplying blood to the kidneys are furred up, less blood is received; the kidneys interpret this as blood pressure being too low, and produce more renin – which causes blood vessels to constrict, and so blood pressure goes up. Even when more blood does arrive, this is processed more slowly due to the reduced number of nephrons present.

New research also suggests that some people develop high blood pressure because they inherit genes that make them less efficient at juggling the regulation of blood pressure and body temperature. This involves directing blood away from internal organs (such as the kidneys) towards the skin, and vice versa. In some people, this juggling effect causes changes within the walls of tiny arteries that lead to hypertension, and renin may be involved. This mechanism is thought to account for 'essential hypertension',

NATURE'S CALL

During youth, the pituitary gland in your brain secretes anti-diuretic hormone (also known as vasopressin) at night, which acts on the kidneys to lower urine production and retain fluid. As the kidneys age, they become less responsive to this signal, so you may need to visit the bathroom more often at night to pass water.

RISK FACTORS:
KIDNEY DISEASE

You are most at risk if you:
- have high blood pressure
- have diabetes
- are overweight
- smoke cigarettes
- have a family history of kidney disease

which tends to run in families and comes on at a relatively young age (in your twenties and thirties).

KIDNEY DISEASE

Kidney disease is often described as 'silent', as it produces few symptoms, though you may notice a change in the frequency and amount of urine you pass, especially at night. Sometimes urine becomes unusually frothy or foaming (due to abnormally high levels of protein leaking into the urine through damaged kidneys), and there may be general puffiness around the eyes and ankles. There may also be discomfort in the kidney area, or when passing urine. As symptoms are often missed, it's a good idea to have an annual urine test to check for signs of hidden protein or blood.

Looking after your kidneys

- **Eat plenty of fruit and vegetables** – these contain potassium, which helps to flush excess sodium salt

Anti-ageing supplements

Antioxidants *such as vitamin C reduce oxidative stress and may help to reduce kidney damage*

Alpha-lipoic acid *(ALA) can reduce oxidative stress and urinary albumin protein excretion (a sign of kidney leakage and damage) in people with diabetes*

Cranberry extracts *help to reduce urinary tract infections*

Dandelion root extracts *are a traditional diuretic, helping to flush excess water from the body*

from the body, which can lower blood pressure.
- **Maintain a healthy weight** and exercise regularly, ideally every day if possible.
- **Check your blood pressure** and blood glucose levels regularly and ensure that they remain well controlled.
- **Keep alcohol intake within recommended limits**, and avoid smoking.
- **Drink enough water** on a daily basis to maintain urine that is a pale straw colour.
- **Reduce stress levels** and have regular relaxation sessions.

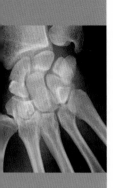

Bones

The most common age-related problem affecting bone is osteoporosis. This develops when not enough new bone is made to replace the old bone that is reabsorbed, so taking steps to improve your bone health is vital.

Although often thought of as inert 'sticks', the 206-plus bones in your body are living tissues made up of a network of collagen fibres filled with mineral salts. These minerals – of which the most important is calcium phosphate – are in a constant state of flux, with new bone continually being made to replace that which is worn out and dissolved away.

Osteoporosis develops when this remodelling activity becomes unbalanced. As a result, bones start to thin, become brittle and fracture more easily.

Looking after your bones

- **Take regular exercise** to stimulate bone formation – at least 30–60 minutes per day. High-impact exercise is best (aerobics, gymnastics, netball, dancing, racket sports, jogging, skipping) but non-weight-bearing exercise such as stretching and swimming is also beneficial. For older people, any form of activity is useful, including walking, climbing stairs, carrying loads, doing housework and gardening. These activities also strengthen muscles to reduce the likelihood of a fall.

RISK FACTORS: OSTEOPOROSIS

- early menopause (before age forty-five) for women, or low levels of testosterone for men
- loss of periods for any cause except pregnancy (for example, excessive dieting/exercise, or use of depot progestogen contraception)
- close-family history – especially if a parent had a hip fracture
- long-term use of high-dose, corticosteroid tablets
- certain medical conditions, such as adrenal, liver or thyroid problems
- being housebound with little exposure to sunlight
- low dietary intakes of magnesium, calcium, phosphorus and vitamin D
- intestinal malabsorption (for instance, due to coeliac disease, Crohn's disease, gastric surgery)
- long-term immobility, especially confinement to bed in childhood
- heavy drinking and/or smoking

- **Obtain good intakes of calcium** throughout life. Sources include dairy products, green leafy vegetables, salmon/pilchards (tinned with bones), eggs, nuts, seeds, pulses, plus white and brown bread made from fortified flour. The easiest way to boost your intake is to drink an extra 500 ml (1 pint) of skimmed or semi-skimmed milk per day, which provides around 720 mg calcium.
- **Get enough vitamin D** – essential for the absorption of calcium from your diet. Just 15 minutes' skin exposure to sunshine when the UV index is greater than 3 can produce vitamin D, but during cold winter months you need to ensure dietary intakes from oily fish, liver, eggs, butter, and fortified milk and margarine/spreads, as well as supplements (*see also* page 93).
- **Eat at least five servings of fruit and veg per day**, as they are rich in vitamins, minerals, antioxidants and isoflavones needed for bone health.
- **Avoid canned, fizzy drinks**, as their high content of phosphoric acid leaches calcium from your bones.
- **Cut back on salty foods** – table salt (sodium chloride) increases the loss of calcium through your kidneys.
- **Avoid smoking cigarettes**, which can lower levels of sex hormones to trigger premature bone-thinning.
- **Avoid aluminium-based antacids**, which impair absorption of phosphates from the gut – regular use for more than ten years may double the risk of a hip fracture.

Anti-ageing supplements

Calcium *and* **phosphate** *for strong bones*

Vitamin D₃ *for optimum calcium absorption from the gut*

Vitamin K₂ *to make osteocalcin, a bone protein that binds calcium*

Magnesium *regulates the flow of calcium in and out of cells and is important for bone strength*

Essential fatty acids *found in evening primrose and fish oils stimulate calcium uptake from the gut, decrease calcium loss in the urine and increase calcium deposition in your bones*

Isoflavones *mimic the beneficial action of oestrogen to increase bone mineralization*

- **Avoid excess stress**, as the stress hormone, cortisol, increases calcium resorption from bone and increases calcium loss in the urine.
- **Consider cutting back on caffeine** – some research suggests those who drink four cups of coffee a day are three times more likely to suffer a hip fracture in later life. To offset this effect, some experts suggest obtaining an extra 40 mg calcium for every 178 ml (6 fl oz) cup of coffee consumed.
- **Avoid heavy consumption of red meat**, as this may reduce absorption of dietary calcium and has been linked with low bone mass and early osteoporosis. Aim to eat meat no more than once a day.

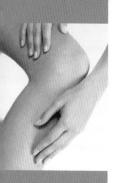

Joints

Your joints undergo significant changes with age and, for many, joint movements become increasingly painful, stiff and restricted. But is there anything you can do help?

There are more than 230 mobile and semi-mobile joints in your body. These are essentially similar, in that their bone ends are covered with slippery articular cartilage, their movements are 'oiled' by synovial fluid and they are held together by strong ligaments.

Synovial fluid becomes thinner and less cushioning as we get older, while articular cartilage becomes softer, stiffer, flaky and less able to withstand compressive forces. In around half of people over the age of sixty, these age-related changes lead to osteoarthritis. The cause is not fully understood, but is believed to result from an active process in which inflammation and an over-zealous healing response result in further loss of cartilage and the formation of bony outgrowths, restricting movement and making it painful.

RISK FACTORS: DETERIORATING JOINTS

Take steps to reduce joint ageing if any of the following apply:

- you are aged forty or over
- arthritis runs in your family
- you are overweight
- you take little exercise
- work or exercise involves repetitive movements of a joint
- you feel the need to stretch your back every day
- you notice creakiness in one or more joints
- your joints are becoming less flexible, swelling, changing shape or aching (especially after exercise)

Looking after your joints

- **Follow a healthy diet** – your joints thrive on the same healthy diet as your heart and brain, with plenty of fresh fruit, vegetables, nuts, seeds, wholegrains and oily fish. Omega-3 fatty acids from oily fish have been shown to reduce the long-term need for painkillers in those with age-related joint problems.
- **Get plenty of vitamin C** – fruit and vegetables are your main dietary source of vitamin C, which is needed for collagen synthesis in cartilage, as well as for its anti-inflammatory antioxidant effects. People with moderate to high intakes of vitamin

Anti-ageing supplements

Omega-3 fish oils *reduce inflammation in joints, to improve pain and swelling*

Glucosamine *has an anti-inflammatory action and stimulates formation of new cartilage and synovial fluids*

Chondroitin *has an anti-inflammatory action and inhibits enzymes that break down cartilage*

Methyl-sulphonyl-methane *(MSM) reduces inflammation, pain and stiffness*

Rosehip extracts *can reduce joint pain and stiffness*

Bromelain *can reduce joint and back pain*

Devil's Claw *has an aspirin-like pain-killing effect on joints*

Ginger *contains a variety of 'warming' substances, such as gingerol and zingerone, which help to reduce joint inflammation*

C are three times less likely to develop knee pain or see their knee osteoarthritis progress than those with low intakes.

- **Maintain a healthy weight** – carrying excess fat increases inflammation in the body as well as the force to which your joints are subjected. For every extra 1 kg (2.2 lb) of weight you carry, the overall force across your knees – when walking or standing – increases by 2–3 kg (4½–6½ lb). So, if you're 10 kg (22 lb) overweight, the force on your knees increases by up to 30 kg (66 lb). Being overweight therefore increases the risk of knee arthritis as much as seven times. Conversely, overweight people who manage to lose 5 kg (11 lb) have been shown to halve their risk of developing of knee osteoarthritis over the following ten years.
- **Exercise daily** to help stimulate joint lubrication and preserve muscle strength. Quality of knee cartilage – in both healthy people and those with osteoarthritis – is directly related to lean muscle mass, and reduces as fat

mass increases. If you're overweight, you therefore need to aim to lose fat without losing muscle – for which exercise is key. The combination of losing body fat and increasing physical activity is more effective for improving pain and physical function in people with osteoarthritis of the knee than either intervention alone.

- **Don't smoke** – people with knee osteoarthritis who smoke are twice as likely to develop cartilage loss and severe knee pain than those who don't smoke, even if they're not overweight.
- **Keep hydrated** – drink sufficient fluids to maintain joint hydration.

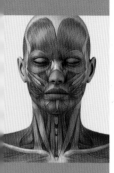

Muscles

If you don't use them, you lose them! As you get older, you lose a significant amount of lean muscle tissue, which is mostly replaced with fat. Reduced energy intake and regular exercise are key to keeping the dreaded middle-age spread at bay ...

Your body contains around 650 voluntary skeletal muscles. In addition, you have innumerable smooth involuntary muscles that perform functions such as controlling the constriction and dilation of blood vessels, and propelling food through your intestines. Arguably your most important muscle, however, is found in your heart, which contains a special type of involuntary striated muscle that beats faithfully every minute of your life.

AGE	KCAL PER DAY	
---	WOMEN	MEN
15–18	2110	2755
19–50	1940	2550
51–59	1900	2550
60–64	1900	2380
65–74	1900	2330
75+	1810	2100

REDUCING YOUR ENERGY INTAKE

Between the ages of twenty-five and seventy, the average woman loses 5 kg (11 lb) of muscle, while the average man loses 10 kg (22 lb). As muscle cells burn more energy than fat, your metabolism slows in proportion to the amount of muscle tissue you have lost. On average, after the age of twenty-five your resting metabolism slows by around 5 per cent every ten years and, as a result, your daily calorie needs also decrease. By the age of seventy-five, a woman needs

around 300 kcal fewer per day than when she was eighteen, and 130 kcal per day fewer than when she was fifty – and the difference is even greater in men (*see* estimated energy requirements above). If you don't reduce your energy intake to compensate for this loss of lean muscle tissue, the inevitable result is middle-age spread.

Looking after your muscles

Exercise every day for at least 30–60 minutes – and, once you are fit, exercise even more. Walking and swimming are particularly beneficial, as these activities involve the action of over 200 muscles without placing excessive strain on ageing joints.

As soon as you start to exercise, blood vessels within contracting muscles dilate to bring in the extra supplies of glucose, fatty acids, oxygen and the minerals and vitamins you need. Regular exercise therefore helps to counterbalance the effects of age to maintain muscle bulk.

Muscle cells obtain energy by burning fuel (glycogen, glucose, fatty acids) within tiny 'factories' called mitochondria. This metabolic activity is one of the main contributors to your resting metabolic rate and calorie needs. Regular exercise increases the number and size of mitochondria present in each 'exercised' muscle cell, so you burn more energy per hour even while you are resting or asleep, thus helping to offset the encroachment of middle-age spread. It also improves insulin resistance and glucose control to protect against the onset of type 2 diabetes.

Anti-ageing supplements

B group vitamins *for the production of energy in muscle cells; vitamin B$_3$ (niacin) is needed by muscle cells to absorb glucose from the circulation*

Antioxidants *(such as vitamins C and E) reduce free-radical damage and have a strengthening effect on muscle fibres*

Magnesium *maintains the electrical stability of muscle cells and is especially important in controlling calcium entry into heart cells to trigger a regular heartbeat*

Co-enzyme Q10 *to process oxygen and generate energy-rich molecules (it's especially important for the increasing number of people taking a statin drug to lower cholesterol; see also page 104)*

Creatine *is a protein-based energy-rich molecule that may help to boost muscle mass*

Conjugated linoleic acid *transports fatty acids away from fatty tissues to muscle cells, where they are burned for fuel (building muscle at the expense of fat)*

HMB (hydroxymethyl butyrate) *is a protein building block that may reduce age-related muscle wasting*

DID YOU KNOW?

Your most powerful muscles are the masseters – chewing muscles which can generate bite pressures of over 120 kg per square centimetre (1,707 lb per square inch) between the teeth.

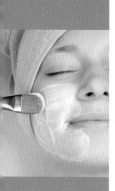

Skin

Your skin forms a waterproof barrier against the outside world, protecting you from physical damage, dehydration and infection, but it's also one of the first parts of the body to show visible signs of ageing.

Our skin helps to control body temperature, makes vitamin D on exposure to sunlight, and contains specialist nerve endings that can detect light touch, sustained pressure, cold, warmth or pain. Many people take their skin for granted, but a little bit of care will reward you with a softer, more youthful outer coat.

QUICK FACTS

- Skin forms the largest organ in your body, with a surface area of up to 2 square metres (21 square feet)
- It has two main layers: an outer epidermis and an inner dermis
- The outer layer is continually being worn away and replaced, as new cells move from the basal layer towards the surface
- You shed around 18 kg (40 lb) of skin during your life
- Household dust is mostly made up of dead skin cells

WRINKLES

The commonest cause of fine lines and wrinkles is over-exposure to sunlight (photo-ageing). There are three main types:

Crinkles: very fine wrinkles that disappear when skin is stretched. These are linked with the breakdown of elastic fibres that starts in the early thirties.

Glyphic wrinkles: accentuations of normal skin lines; skin becomes thickened and yellow in tone, especially where exposed to sunlight (such as around the eyes, and on the neck and backs of hands).

Linear furrows: deepening of the normal grooves related to facial expressions; the positions of these are determined very early in life.

Wearing sunscreen is one of the most effective ways to reduce premature skin ageing (*see* opposite), but there are a number of other things you can do to help, too.

PRIMROSE POWER

In one trial involving forty women, with an average age of forty-four, those taking 3 g evening primrose oil daily experienced a 20 per cent improvement in skin moisture, smoothness, elasticity and firmness.

Looking after your skin

- **Follow a healthy, wholegrain diet** supplying at least five servings of fruit and vegetables and a handful of nuts/seeds daily, plus fish two or three times a week. As skin cells turn over so rapidly, lack of vitamins, minerals and essential fatty acids can quickly lead to problems such as dryness, flakiness, dullness, pimples and premature wrinkles.
- **Drink plenty of water** – at least 2.5 litres (around 5 pints) a day. Fluids are important for skin hydration and suppleness.
- **Cleanse, tone and moisturize** your skin twice daily, using good-quality skin-care products.

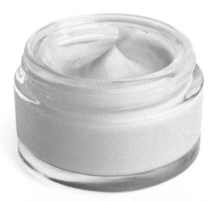

Anti-ageing supplements

Evening primrose *and* **borage oils** *improve dryness and suppleness*

Omega-3 fish oils *improve skin lustre and have an inflammatory action to help improve itching, redness and scaling*

Green tea *contains powerful flavonoid antioxidants, which help to protect against premature skin ageing*

Vitamin E *is a powerful antioxidant which, because it is fat-soluble, protects skin from oxidation*

Vitamin C *for synthesis of collagen (in addition to its antioxidant properties), an important structural protein in skin*

Co-enzyme Q10 *is added to some skin creams to reduce premature wrinkles*

- **Avoid excessive exposure to the sun** and *never* use tanning beds.
- **Always wear sun protection products** containing both UVA and UVB sunscreens. Wear sunscreen with a sun protection factor of at least SPF8 when going outdoors in winter; during summer, products with SPF30 will protect against the leading cause of premature skin ageing: ultraviolet radiation (*see also* pages 90–92).
- **Avoid smoking** (active and passive) – smokers are five times more likely to develop premature wrinkles than non-smokers.

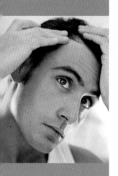

Hair

While you might not be able to beat genetic hair loss, there is much that can be done to keep hair follicles healthy, and combat the hair loss and thinning that naturally occurs with age.

We each have between 100,000 and 150,000 hair follicles on our head, with blondes tending to have more than brunettes. Each hair has its own life cycle, growing vigorously for up to six years (anagen phase) followed by a resting period (catagen phase) of 3–6 months. While resting, the hair root shrinks, loosens and eventually falls out (telogen phase), as the hair follicle reactivates to produce a new hair shaft.

Because each hair has its own cycle, we lose around 80–100 scalp hairs per day. If daily losses are greater than this, gradual thinning occurs, especially in later life, when hair growth slows.

BALDNESS

The most common hair problem associated with age is male-pattern baldness (androgenic alopecia), which can affect women as well as men. This form of diffuse hair loss over the top of the scalp is often genetic, passing down through the female line. It is believed to result from increased activity of 5-alpha reductase, an enzyme which converts testosterone hormone into dihydrotestosterone in scalp-hair follicles. This acts as the signal for the production of progressively finer hairs

with each new growth cycle, before follicles eventually lie dormant.

HEALTH GAUGE

Your hair is a good indicator of your general health and nutrition. It's often the first part of your body to show signs of ill health, or a dietary lack of vitamins, minerals or essential fatty acids. This is because, although hair is often thought of as a dead structure, its root – the hair follicle – is very

DID YOU KNOW?

After the age of twenty-five, the diameter of individual hairs naturally reduces, especially in women. Although this often goes unnoticed, it can change the texture and body of your hair. By the age of forty, most people have finer hair with less body. At the same time, more follicles stay in their resting phase, so less hair grows and the rate of growth decreases, resulting in progressive thinning.

much alive. The rate at which new hair cells are produced is second only to the speed at which new blood cells are made in the bone marrow. Your hair follicles therefore need a constant supply of nutrients for optimum health. Unlike the marrow, however, hair is a non-essential structure and your body preferentially diverts precious nutrient stores away from it in times of lack or stress.

Looking after your hair

- **Eat a healthy, balanced diet** containing as many unrefined wholefoods as possible, especially wholegrains, fruit, vegetables, nuts and seeds for vitamins, minerals and essential fatty acids.
- **Don't eat erratically,** crash diet or skip meals, especially breakfast. Eat something at least every four hours (a healthy snack such as fresh or dried fruit, for example).
- **Aim to eat a source of protein**, such as poultry, fish, eggs, nuts or beans, with every meal; hair contains a tough, fibrous protein, keratin, which is made from amino-acid building blocks obtained from your diet.
- **Reduce your salt intake** – excess salt reduces hair-follicle function, and research shows that reducing salt intake can reduce hair loss and thinning by as much as 60 per cent.
- **Stimulate blood flow to hair follicles** by massaging your scalp regularly with your fingers, ideally on most

days. Hold handfuls of hair near the roots and move the scalp back and forth and from side to side, to help loosen underlying tightness.
- **Try to avoid excess stress**, as stress hormones constrict blood supply to the scalp and hair follicles, reducing their supply of nutrients. This can lead to generalized hair-thinning or even patchy hair loss. If you are stressed, your scalp will tighten; use massage and scalp movement to loosen it and improve circulation to hair follicles.
- **Keep a positive outlook** on life, as negative thoughts have a profound effect on your overall health and that of rapidly dividing cells, such as those in your hair follicles.

Anti-ageing supplements

An A-to-Z-style multivitamin and mineral *as a nutritional safety net*

Omega-3 fish oils *to improve hair texture and shine*

Evening primrose oil *to improve skin and hair suppleness*

Silica *(for example, from bamboo or herbal horsetail), found in hair, skin and nail supplements, to boost hair-shaft strength*

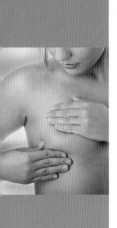

Breasts

Breast cancer remains the most frequently occurring cancer in women, and, while the majority of breast lumps are benign, the earlier diagnosis is made, the better. Regular monitoring to check for breast changes is therefore crucial.

One in three women will discover a breast lump at some time during their life. Although most of these are benign fibroadenomas (fibrous glandular masses) or fluid-filled cysts, overall, one in eight women will eventually develop breast cancer, and a small number of men are also affected. The earlier the diagnosis is made, the more likely it is that treatment will result in a cure. For this reason, women are advised to be aware of how their breasts normally feel, so they can easily detect changes; 90 per cent of breast lumps are discovered by women or their partners.

POSSIBLE CAUSES

The cause of breast cancer is still poorly understood, as known risk factors only explain a small proportion of cases. These risk factors include a close-family history of breast cancer (such as mother or sister), having a first child after the age of thirty, never having had children, not breast-feeding, early onset of periods (aged twelve or younger) and late menopause. Other factors that have been linked with an increased risk of breast cancer include being obese, drinking excessive amounts of alcohol, smoking cigarettes and eating a diet that is high in fat (especially animal fat) and low in fruit,

BREAST-CANCER CHECK POINTS

Some breasts are naturally more lumpy than others, and breasts may also change at different times of your monthly cycle. By learning how they feel at different times, however, subtle changes can be detected. Check them when in the bath or shower, or when dressing. If you notice any changes, seek medical advice straight away.

- **Examine** your breasts regularly.
- **Get to know** their normal look and feel.
- **Look out for** any lumps, dimpling, thickening or change in shape and size.
- **Attend** regular breast-screening mammography when invited.

You can create your own Early Detection Plan at www.nationalbreastcancer.org.

Anti-ageing supplements

Antioxidants *help to neutralize free radicals, which are linked with premature ageing*

Omega-3 fish oils *provide building blocks that have a beneficial effect on hormone balance*

Soy isoflavones – *several studies show that women with the highest intake of isoflavones are half as likely to develop breast cancer as women with a lower intake; isoflavones are believed to block oestrogen receptors in the breasts to reduce the effects of stronger human oestrogens*

vegetables and fibre. These factors either increase your risk of inheriting a gene linked with breast cancer, or increase your lifetime exposure to the female hormone oestrogen. Many breast tumour cells contain oestrogen receptors that seem to stimulate tumour growth, although not all breast cancers are hormone-dependent.

Looking after your breasts

- **Follow a low-fat, high-fibre diet** – in particular, cut back on your intake of saturated (animal) fats.
- **Eat at least five servings of fruit and vegetables daily** for antioxidants and fibre. Some plant foods contain substances that protect against cancer, such as isoflavones (for example, soybeans), limonene (citrus), sulphoraphane (broccoli) and ellagic acid (berries).
- **Eat more oily fish** – essential fatty acids found in fish oils have been shown to halt the growth of some cancer cells.

- **Lose any excess weight** – fatty tissues can make oestrogen from other circulating hormones.
- **Take regular brisk exercise** – at least 30–60 minutes on most days.
- **Avoid excess alcohol**, as this boosts the effects of oestrogen. Some research suggests that just drinking one unit of alcohol per day increases the risk of breast cancer by 11 per cent, two units daily increases it by 24 per cent, while three units daily may increase the risk by 38 per cent. Sadly, it does not seem that red wine, for all its antioxidant properties, is protective against breast cancer.
- **Don't smoke cigarettes** – a review of thirteen studies found that women who smoke are 20–50 per cent more likely to develop breast cancer than those who don't.

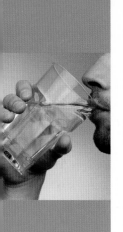

Bladder

The most common age-related problem in this area is urinary incontinence, but pelvic floor exercises can do wonders – both for prevention as well as treatment.

Your bladder is an elastic, muscular sac that can stretch to hold over 500 ml (1 pint) of fluid. Urinary incontinence, however, tends to become more common as we get older, although it can affect people of any age; it's also more common in women than in men (mainly due to childbirth, but also due to the anatomy of the pelvic floor). Some cases are due to weakness of the pelvic floor muscles (known as stress urinary incontinence, on exertion, coughing or sneezing), while others are linked with overactivity of bladder-wall muscles (urge urinary incontinence), or both together (mixed urinary incontinence), in which involuntary leakage is associated with both urgency and also physical stress. Infections and problems affecting the nervous system may also play a role.

PELVIC FLOOR EXERCISES

Exercise 1 Hold in the muscles of your front and back passages as if trying not to go to the toilet. Tighten these muscles upwards once, twice, three times, as if they are an elevator rising and stopping at three floors. Hold for a count of four before letting go. When you return to the normal position, push the muscles out, then tighten up the pelvic floor again. If you find it easy to hold for a count of four, try to hold for longer – up to 10 seconds.

Exercise 2 Lie, stand or sit with your knees slightly apart. Slowly tighten and pull up your pelvic floor muscles as hard as you can. Hold for as long as possible, then relax slowly. Rest for about 10 seconds in between each contraction. Repeat five to ten times.

Exercise 3 Lie, stand or sit with your knees slightly apart. Pull up the muscles hard, then relax immediately. Repeat five to ten times. As your muscles become stronger, hold the contraction for longer and do more pull-ups.

Anti-ageing supplements

Cranberry extracts *help to prevent urinary tract infections*

Probiotics *may help to reduce the occurrence of urinary tract infections*

Isoflavones *have a natural oestrogen-like action for those preferring not to take HRT*

Exercises to strengthen the pelvic floor muscles (the broad sling of muscle stretching from the pubic bone in the front to the base of the tail bone at the rear, forming the floor of the pelvis) are often helpful for both prevention and treatment (*see* left).

STRENGTHENING YOUR PELVIC FLOOR

A minimum of eight pelvic floor muscle contractions should be performed at least three times a day. Quality, rather than quantity, is the key. Although it may sound easy, the trick is to squeeze and lift these muscles *without* pulling in your stomach, squeezing your legs together, tightening your buttocks or holding your breath.

To check you are training the right muscles, sit on the toilet with your legs apart and stop your urinary flow without moving your legs or squeezing your buttocks. If you can do it, you are tightening the right muscles (only do this to learn the technique, however; if you do it regularly, you could cause an infection). You may find it helpful to place a hand on your abdomen, to check it stays relaxed while performing the exercises. Progressive resistance vaginal training devices and electrical pelvic muscle stimulators are also available.

Pull in your pelvic floor muscles before coughing, sneezing or lifting, and avoid standing for long periods of time.

Looking after your bladder

- **Drink sufficient fluids** to maintain straw-coloured urine.
- **Avoid caffeinated drinks**, as caffeine may irritate the bladder. Strong coffee (espresso) also has a diuretic effect; this effect is less obvious with tea, as it is offset by the fluid present in the drink.
- **Remain physically fit** – many forms of exercise have a toning effect on pelvic muscles.
- **Perform pelvic floor exercises** every day, to strengthen the muscles and keep them toned.
- **Maintain a healthy weight** to avoid straining pelvic floor muscles – especially if you tend to put on weight around the waist.

Prostate

The prostate gland often enlarges from middle age onwards, resulting in a variety of symptoms with increasing age, but prostate health can be improved through your diet ...

The prostate is a male gland that lies just beneath the bladder, wrapped around the urinary tube (urethra). After the age of forty-five, the number of cells in the prostate often increases and the gland starts to enlarge. Why this happens is not fully understood, but it's linked with the conversion of the male hormone, testosterone, to a more powerful hormone, dihydrotestosterone, which triggers division of prostate cells. This is known as benign prostatic hyperplasia (BPH). Half of all sixty-year-old men are affected and, by the age of eighty, four out of five men have evidence of BPH.

SYMPTOMS OF AN ENLARGED PROSTATE

Enlargement of the prostate squeezes the urinary tube to interfere with urinary flow. Typical symptoms include:

- difficulty starting to pass water (hesitancy)
- a weak urinary stream
- having to strain to pass water
- starting and stopping when passing water
- dribbling of urine after voiding
- urinary discomfort
- having to rush to the toilet to pass water (urgency)
- having to pass water more often (frequency)
- having to get up at night to pass water (nocturia)
- a feeling of not having emptied the bladder fully

Symptoms are not always linked to prostate size, as it can expand outwards without squeezing the urethra, so if you experience any of the above on an ongoing basis visit your doctor.

QUICK FACTS

- The prostate produces secretions that nourish sperm, and acts like a valve to prevent ejaculation backwards into the bladder
- It's the size and shape of a large chestnut during your twenties ...
- ... the size of an apricot during your forties ...
- ... and can reach the size of a lemon in your sixties (or, occasionally, the size of a grapefruit, although this is rare)

Anti-ageing supplements

Zinc *helps to regulate prostate sensitivity to hormones*

Lycopene *has a protective effect on prostate cell division*

Soy isoflavones *have been linked with improved prostate health*

Saw palmetto *may reduce conversion of testosterone to dihydrotestosterone, helping the central part of an enlarged gland to shrink*

Evening primrose oil *contains essential fatty acids that are beneficial to prostate health*

Looking after your prostate

The prostate thrives on the same healthy diet recommended for heart health.

- **Follow a diet low in saturated (animal) fat** and eat at least five servings of fresh fruit or vegetables per day for vitamins, minerals and antioxidants. In particular, select more Japanese-style foods, as weak plant hormones (phytoestrogens) found in soy products and other Asian vegetables such as beansprouts, Chinese leaves, bok choy (pak choi) and kohlrabi help to discourage prostate gland enlargement.
- **Eat a high-fibre diet**, which binds male hormones in the gut that have been flushed out through the bile, to reduce their reabsorption.
- **Select zinc-rich foods** such as seafood (especially oysters), wholegrains, bran, pumpkin seeds, garlic and pulses, as zinc is important for prostate health and controls its sensitivity to hormones.
- **Eat plenty of tomatoes** and tomato-based foods – these contain lycopene and other carotenoids that can protect against prostate cancer.
- **Eat plenty of nuts and seeds** – these contain essential fatty acids needed to make prostaglandins (hormone-like substances important for prostate health).

Tomatoes can help protect against prostate cancer.

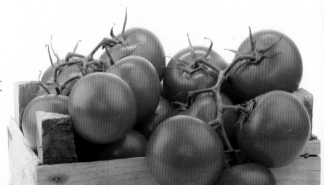

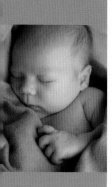

Fertility

Women reach a biological fertility cut-off at the menopause, but recent research suggests that men also need to keep an eye on their biological clock if they wish to father a child.

While men can, in theory, father a child from puberty throughout the rest of their life, analysis of male patients at an infertility clinic suggests their chance of success reduces by 7 per cent per year between the ages of forty-one and forty-five, and falls more sharply among older men. This is because the quality of sperm deteriorates with age. A study involving men aged twenty-two to eighty years found that semen volume falls by 0.03 ml per year, sperm motility falls by 0.7 per cent per year, and the ability of sperm to swim forwards reduces by 4.7 per cent a year.

Women, on the other hand, possess around half a million eggs at the time of puberty, but these disappear or stop responding to hormone signals at a rate of 1,000–1,500 per month. Eventually, at the average age of fifty-one, the female menopause is triggered as the ovaries run out of eggs. Oestrogen levels start to fall before this time,

FERTILITY TESTS

• **FOR MEN**, semen analysis will show whether or not sperm quality and quantity are within normal limits of:

Volume: greater than 2.0 ml
Concentration: greater than 20 million/ml
Total cells: greater than 40 million
Motility: greater than 50 per cent
Normal forms: greater than 14 per cent

• **FOR WOMEN**, a blood test to measure levels of Anti-Müllerian Hormones (AMH) can assess how many eggs remain in the ovaries (ovarian reserve). This is important information for women who are planning to postpone childbirth into their thirties or forties. The results will show whether or not this is a wise decision. Typical results are as follows:

	AMH concentration pmol/L
Optimal fertility:	28.6–48.5
Satisfactory fertility:	15.7–28.6
Low fertility:	2.2–15.7
Very low fertility:	0.0–2.2

Anti-ageing supplements

A multivitamin and mineral *as a nutritional safety net*

Antioxidants *(vitamin C, vitamin E, selenium) to protect sperm cells from damage*

Zinc *for the function of sex hormones, and to prevent premature release of chemicals in the sperm head needed to drill through the egg during fertilization*

Folic acid *is essential for normal cell division, including sperm production and early pregnancy*

along with fertility, so that a woman aged twenty-five years, for example, may become pregnant within two or three months of trying, while for a woman aged thirty-five it can take between six months and two years – or longer – to conceive.

Looking after your fertility

- **Eat a healthy diet** supplying at least five servings of fruit and vegetables per day – and preferably eight to ten, if you can manage it.
- **Maintain a healthy weight**, as being overweight affects hormone balance, insulin resistance and glucose control, all of which impact fertility.
- **Exercise regularly** – this can boost fertility by improving insulin resistance and glucose control.
- **Have a sexual health check-up** at a sexual health clinic. Some sexually transmissible infections such as chlamydia may cause few symptoms but can reduce fertility.
- **Stop smoking** – women who smoke ten or more cigarettes per day are three times more likely to experience difficulty in conceiving than non-

smokers, while male smokers are only half as fertile as non-smokers.
- **Avoid alcohol**, as it acts as a cell poison. Women who drink five or fewer units of alcohol per week are twice as likely to conceive within six months as those drinking ten units or more per week. Forty per cent of male sub-fertility is linked with alcohol intake (even at moderate consumption).
- **Avoid excess stress**, as this can affect fertility by lowering levels of sex hormones.
- **Use an ovulation predictor kit** to pinpoint the fertile period and optimize your chances of conception, as the timing of ovulation is extremely unpredictable, especially in older women.

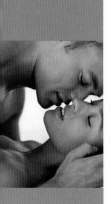

Sexual function

Low sex drive is by far the most common age-related problem when it comes to sexual issues. But don't despair – there are things you can do to help.

Although erection difficulties affect an estimated one in ten adult males, low sex drive is the most widespread problem affecting us as we age – and the number one reason for visiting a sex therapist. Surveys suggest that loss of libido affects 30 per cent of middle-aged and 72 per cent of post-menopausal women, with 60 per cent of men experiencing stress and 45 per cent of those with enlarged-prostate symptoms also being affected.

HORMONE LEVELS

Testosterone is the main hormone that controls libido in both men and women. Although most men don't experience a menopause-like drop in sex-hormone levels, low testosterone levels develop in around 7 per cent of men aged forty to sixty, 20 per cent of men aged sixty to eighty, and 35 per cent of men over eighty.

As with low oestrogen levels in women, low testosterone levels (sometimes

ADAM QUESTIONNAIRE	YES	NO
1 Do you have a decreased libido (sex drive)	☐	☐
2 Do you have a lack of energy?	☐	☐
3 Do you have a decrease in strength and/or endurance?	☐	☐
4 Have you lost height?	☐	☐
5 Have you noticed a decreased 'enjoyment of life'?	☐	☐
6 Are you sad and/or grumpy?	☐	☐
7 Are your erections less strong?	☐	☐
8 Have you noticed a recent deterioration in your ability to play sports?	☐	☐
9 Are you falling asleep after dinner?	☐	☐
10 Has there been a recent deterioration in your work performance?	☐	☐

If you answered yes to question 1 or 7, or any three other questions, you may have testosterone deficiency syndrome. Talk to your doctor to have your testosterone levels checked.

referred to as andropause) are linked with male symptoms of tiredness, irritability, lowered sex drive, aching joints, dry skin, insomnia, excessive sweating, hot flushes and depression.

If you're male and aged forty or over, find out whether you could have low testosterone levels by taking the ADAM (Androgen Deficiency in Aging Males) questionnaire, developed by an endocrinologist from the St Louis University School of Medicine (*see* left).

Looking after your libido

- **Consider hormone replacement therapy.** Appropriate use of oestrogen and testosterone replacement therapy in women and men respectively can boost libido and overcome many of the age-related metabolic changes (insulin resistance, poor glucose control, high blood pressure, abnormal cholesterol levels) associated with loss of sex hormones. In addition, testosterone replacement therapy can improve erectile problems in 60 per cent of cases – and having a normal testosterone level increases the chance of a good response to impotence drugs such as sildenafil. Visit your doctor for advice.

Anti-ageing supplements

St John's Wort *can improve sex drive as well as mood in post-menopausal women*

Catuaba *promotes erotic dreams, followed by increased sexual desire within three weeks of regular treatment*

Damiana *can promote desire, by increasing blood flow and nerve sensitivity in the genitals*

Muira Puama *stimulates desire through direct action on brain chemicals*

Ginkgo biloba *increases blood flow to improve erectile function*

Ginseng *increases levels of nitric oxide in the spongy tissue of the penis and clitoris (an effect similar to that of erectile drugs such as sildenafil)*

Soy isoflavones *can boost oestrogen levels in women*

Zinc *extracts help to maintain testosterone levels in both men and women*

- **Stop smoking and cut back on alcohol,** as this can significantly boost sex hormone levels in both men and pre-menopausal women.
- **Get some sun!** Research suggests that men who expose their chest to sunlight experience a 120 per cent rise in circulating testosterone levels, which persists for several days – and levels increased by 200 per cent when the genital area was exposed.
- **Try a lubricant** – using an intimate lubricant will overcome dryness and reduce the discomfort experienced by some menopausal women during sex.

RESOURCES

HEART AND CIRCULATORY HEALTH

American Heart Association
www.americanheart.org

American Society of Hypertension
www.ash-us.org

American Stroke Association
www.strokeassociation.org

Blood Pressure Association (UK)
www.bpassoc.org.uk

British Heart Foundation
www.bhf.org.uk

Heart Foundation of Australia
www.heartfoundation.com.au

Heart Foundation of New Zealand
www.heartfoundation.org.nz

Heart and Stroke Foundation of Canada
www.heartandstroke.ca

Heart UK – The Cholesterol Charity
www.heartuk.org.uk

Hypertension Canada
www.hypertension.ca

HEALTHY DIET

Academy of Nutrition and Dietetics (formerly American Dietetic Association)
www.eatright.org

British Dietetic Association
www.bda.uk.com

British Nutrition Foundation
www.nutrition.org.uk

Dietitians Association of Australia
www.daa.asn.au

Dieticians of Canada
www.dieticians.ca

Dietitians NZ
www.dietitians.org.nz

Glycemic Index (home of)
www.glycemicindex.com

The Nutrition Society (UK)
www.nutritionsociety.org

US Department of Agriculture's Food and Nutrition Information Center
www.nutrition.gov

SMOKING

Action on Smoking and Health Australia
www.ashaust.org.au

Action on Smoking and Health Canada
www.ash.ca

Action on Smoking and Health UK
www.ash.org.uk

Action on Smoking and Health US
www.ash.org

The Foundation for a Smokefree America
www.anti-smoking.org

Quit UK
www.quit.org.uk

Smokefree NZ
www.smokefree.co.nz

COMPLEMENTARY MEDICINE ASSOCIATIONS

Australian Traditional-Medicine Society
www.atms.com.au

British Complementary Medicine Association
www.bcma.co.uk

New Zealand Natural Medicine Association
www.nznma.com

US National Center for Complementary and Alternative Medicine
www.nccam.nih.gov

OTHER RECOMMENDED TITLES
by Dr Sarah Brewer

Death: A Survival Guide, Quercus, 2011

Cut Your Stress, Quercus, 2010

Essential Guide to Vitamins, Minerals and Herbal Supplements,
Right Way, 2010

The Human Body, Quercus, 2009

Cut Your Cholesterol, Quercus, 2009

Low-Cholesterol Cookbook for Dummies,
Wiley, 2009

Natural Health Guru: Overcoming Arthritis, Duncan Baird, 2009

Natural Health Guru: Overcoming Asthma, Duncan Baird, 2009

Natural Health Guru: Overcoming High Blood Pressure, Duncan Baird, 2008

Natural Health Guru: Overcoming Diabetes, Duncan Baird, 2008

Menopause for Dummies, Wiley, 2007

Thyroid for Dummies, Wiley, 2006

Arthritis for Dummies, Wiley, 2006

Natural Approaches to Diabetes,
Piatkus, 2005

Intimate Relations: Living and Loving in Later Life, Age Concern, 2004

The Total Detox Plan,
Carlton, 2000, 2011

INDEX

PICTURE CREDITS

Cover (from top left, in rows): iStockphoto: Christine Keene/Hugo Chang/Linda Alstead/Michael Courtney/ Joan Vicent Cantó Roig/Mojca Kobal/Pali Rao/Rami Halim/Angelika Schwarz/JackJelly/Charlotte Allen/ Mark Wragg/Pascal Genest/Studio-Annika/Jacob Wackerhausen; Flickr: Alex Bramwell; iStockphoto: Jill Chen/Mercè Bellera/Supermimicry; Image Source: David Cleveland

Image Source 12–13 OJO Images; 15 Fancy; 21 Cultura RF; 24b SPL; 26b Photolibrary; 27 Corbis RF; 31 Clover; 33 Fancy; 38 Food Collection; 47 OJO Images; 48 Jamie Beck; 51 Food Collection; 53 Fancy; 55 Ablelmages; 69r OJO Images; 71 Food Collection; 72–73; 81; 82 OJO Images; 85 Henry Arden; 87 Jose Luis Pelaez, Inc; 89 Cultura RF; 91; 95; 102 (&5) David Cleveland; 108–109; 119b Jose Luis Pelaez, Inc; 132 SPL; 134

iStockphoto 14 (&4) Christine Keene; 19 Joe Biafore; 20 (&4) Hugo Chang; 24t (&4) Linda Alstead; 25 martinturzak; 29 Donald Erickson; 30 (&4) Michael Courtney; 34t (&4) Joan Vicent Cantó Roig; 35tl,tr,br Cristian Baitg; 37 Magdalena Marczewska; 40 (&5) Mojca Kobal; 41 Lauri Patterson; 46 (&5) Pali Rao; 50 (&5) Rami Halim; 54 (&5) Angelika Schwarz; 58 (&5) JackJelly; 59 Elena Elisseeva; 62t (&4) Charlotte Allen; 66 (&4) Mark Wragg; 72t (&4) Pascal Genest; 75 Arpad Benedek; 76t (&4) Studio-Annika; 77 Knape; 80 (&4) Jacob Wackerhausen; 90t (&5) Jill Chen; 94t (&5) Mercè Bellera; 96 Jacob Wackerhausen; 98 (&5) Supermimicry; 110 Enrico Fianchini; 111, 113, 115, 117t, 119t, 121t, 123, 125t, 127, 129, 131, 133, 135, 137, 139t, 141t, 143t, 145, 147, 149t, 151, 153 Dovile Butvilaite; 125b Marcela Barsse

Shutterstock.com 6–11 Elaine Barker; 16 LianeM; 17, 18, 26t, 34b, 38b, 49, 52, 62b, 69l, 73tr, 76b, 90b, 94b, 97, 100 Kellis; 22 photosync; 22–23 PeJo; 44 Svetlana Lukienko; 56 nice_pictures; 61 Johan Swanepoel; 63 Skyline; 64–5 Kuzmin Andrey; 78 Lasse Kristensen; 99 AISPIX by Image Source; 101 Elena Schweitzer; 103 foto76; 105 Monkey Business Images; 106 kukuruxa; 112 Yakobchuk Vasy; 114 AISPIX by Image Source; 116 Ivanova Inga; 117b Nico Tucol; 118 Brian A Jackson; 120 Ariwasabi; 121b Mike Tan C.T; 122 Roger Jegg; 124 kuleczka; 126 Sebastian Kaulitzki; 126–7 spilman; 128 Alexander Raths; 130 Netfalls-Remy Musser; 136 Oleksii Abramov; 138 CLIPAREA/Custom media; 139b Lucie Lang; 140 Glovatskiy; 141b maryo; 142 Diego Cervo; 143b artproem; 144 Piotr Marcinski; 146 Alex Advertising Photography; 148 Christophe Testi; 149b Peter Zijlstra; 150 Denis Kukareko; 152 Yuri Arcurs

Miscellaneous 43 Steve Baxter/Digital Vision/Getty Images; 84 (&5) Alex Bramwell/Flickr

A CONNECTIONS EDITION

This edition published in Great Britain in 2012 by Connections Book Publishing Limited St Chad's House, 148 King's Cross Road London WC1X 9DH www.connections-publishing.com

Text copyright © Dr Sarah Brewer 2012
This edition copyright © Eddison Sadd Editions 2012

British Library Cataloguing-in-Publication data available on request.

ISBN 978-1-85906-345-3

10 9 8 7 6 5 4 3 2 1

Phototypeset in Benton Gothic, Life and Weidemann using InDesign on Apple Macintosh Printed in China

ACKNOWLEDGEMENTS

I would like to thank everyone who has been so helpful in providing research papers and information for the insights explored in this book.

EDDISON•SADD EDITIONS

Creative Director Nick Eddison
Editorial Director Ian Jackson
Managing Editor Tessa Monina
Proofreader Nikky Twyman
Indexer Marie Lorimer
Designer Jane McKenna
Picture research administration Rosie Taylor
Production Sarah Rooney